I HOPE I GET WELL

I HOPE I GET WELL

I HOPE I GET WELL

— A Memoir of Bipolar Disorder —

Adam Gerhardstein

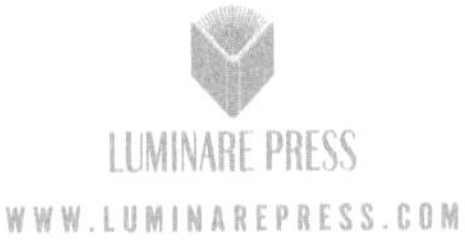

LUMINARE PRESS

WWW.LUMINAREPRESS.COM

Luminare Press
442 Charnelton St.
Eugene, OR 97401
www.luminarepress.com

LCCN: 2024905137
ISBN: 979-8-88679-519-6

"Daddy, who are you going to dedicate your book to?" Phoenix asks with a grin.

I smile at her and put my fork down. "I think I know who you want me to dedicate it to."

My six-year-old beams. "I could be famous!"

My wife, Meredith, and I chuckle, and I tell her I'll think about it.

The next night, back at the dinner table, Phoenix says, "Daddy, I have a new idea for who you should dedicate your book to."

"Oh, yeah. Who?"

"What is the disease you have again called?" she asks. I look up from my plate. "Bipolar disorder."

"Yes, you could dedicate it to all the people with bipolar disorder who I hope will get well."

Chapter 1

SEPTEMBER 23, 2022

St. Paul, Minnesota

I asked for this meeting, but now I can't find the words. We are seated in the school office, and I'm looking down at my shoes, shaking my head. "I don't know what to do," I say. "I'm really trying, but…"

I take a deep breath and fall silent.

My boss says supportive things, gives me ideas, and offers help, but I can tell by her tone that she's worried about her hire.

Who have I become?

When I was a part-time assistant teacher, I had patience. I was gentle and kind, playful and warm. The young children loved me. My supervising teacher called one of my three-year-old students my barnacle—she never left my side. But that was at a different school in another job.

Here, as a full-time lead teacher, I've turned into an irritable, short-tempered jerk. Only one month in, and I've been yelling at kids, grabbing them when they misbehave, and sending them to the office. I can't even get them out to the playground without losing a child along the way.

My boss doesn't know it, but I've been coming home drained—my mind racing, unable to fall asleep.

I bring my hands to my face and rub my temples.

Finally, I meet her eyes. "I'm struggling."

On my bike ride home, I observe myself—my body is taut, my mood erratic, and my thoughts are feral. I let out a moan. It's bad.

Meredith hugs me soon after I walk in the door. She must sense my dread. I tell her what I'm considering, and she hugs me again, this time longer and stronger. We talk. And then I go outside, look up at the sky, and take out my phone.

I tell my boss I need the next week off, that I have bipolar disorder and I'm not feeling well.

After hanging up, I stand in our backyard—my energy stolen, my mind suddenly blank, and my spirit slapped. *What now?*

As I lay in bed that night, a devastating thought hits me. I inspect it, pick it apart from every angle, try to avoid it, and bury it, but it persists.

Is it possible I might not be able to work full-time ever again?

My thoughts spiral from there.

Has my bipolar disorder gotten worse? Have I weakened? Have I become disabled? Have I been disabled all along?

I think through all my years of full-time work since my diagnosis eighteen years ago. I explored four different career paths, and each field held promise. But when I finally chose Montessori education and began my training, I thought I had found my calling.

During my first year, I worked mornings as an assistant at my daughter Phoenix's school. I fell in love with my students and savored every moment. But in my second year, when I tried to work full days to fill in for an assistant teacher who abruptly quit, it triggered my bipolar disorder, and I dropped back down to part-time.

After finishing my training, I received so much encouragement from my instructors that I convinced myself I could learn from and overcome the difficulties I had working full-time. So, I decided to make the leap to a full-time lead teacher.

Now I am one month in, yelling at three-year-olds, unable to sleep, thoughts perseverating, and giant waves of emotion crashing over me.

I wake before Meredith, and I'm sitting on our kitchen stool when she comes downstairs. Phoenix is in the living room, wearing her headphones, watching the TV series *Wild Kratts* on our iPad. Meredith makes her coffee as normal, but when she looks at me, she senses something is terribly wrong.

"What's going on?"

When I open my mouth to answer, the pain of failure and the pain of being bipolar makes it hard to speak. Years of questioning, tension, and momentary self-doubt overwhelm me.

"I don't think…I can work…full-time ever again," I say between sobs.

Meredith's own eyes well with tears as she wraps her arms around me and holds me as I rock back and forth. I feel an emptying, and my overflowing tears bring on a flood of memories—all the times I've struggled in my pursuits, had to take a mental health day, ask for more time to do an assignment, and ask to work fewer hours. Throughout it all, I've told myself I can do anything, that bipolar disorder won't limit me. I can manage it and still do big things. And I have…until I can't.

Two years of training, two years of loving being a teacher, and two years of thinking about how I would run my own classroom. And now, one month in, I know deep in my heart I cannot do it. I can't work full-time as a teacher and manage my bipolar disorder at the same time. Not now, perhaps never, and it's breaking my heart because I love being a teacher.

My future looks empty. All my ambitions as a Montessorian appear unattainable. Where a week earlier I saw unlimited possibilities, I now see no path forward.

I need help.

I called this therapist because her office is within walking distance of our house, and she has good reviews on Google. She happened to have an opening on Tuesday.

So here I am, having wept uncontrollably a few days ago, in agony over whether to leave my new job and what that may mean for my future.

Before I can explain all of this to Dr. Fossum, I know she needs some background, so I launch into an abbreviated version of my mental health history. My diagnosis when I was a college student in Cincinnati, Ohio. How it started with a manic episode and hospitalization, followed by a long depression.

I tell her about my recovery and my decision to move away from Cincinnati. I explain how I've managed my illness since then. How I'm mostly stable. But when I feel some hypomania or a bout of depression coming on, I confine myself in my room with an adventure novel, a streaming device, all my comfort foods, and zone out, give it time, and wait for the pressure of my illness to release.

I tell her this proudly—it's the treatment I devised, and so far, it's worked. For the last sixteen years, I haven't had a full-blown manic episode, been hospitalized, or had a prolonged depression.

"There's a time for distraction," Dr. Fossum says.

I stare at her in silence. Dr. Thyra Fossum. She says it as if it's so obvious, as if, of course, I've always known what I've been doing is distracting myself. She says it as if there's another way to handle the difficult parts of being bipolar.

Distraction.

Is that what I've been doing all these years? When bipolar disorder has flared up and when I've hit a rough patch, have I just been avoiding it? Escaping?

The questions don't take long to answer. Almost as soon as her words register, my story cracks, and my pride retreats. I know it's true. Every single time bipolar disorder has made itself known, I've grown silent, withdrawn into myself, and privately panicked that the worst might be happening again.

"Well, that's how I've been dealing with bipolar disorder since I left Cincinnati sixteen years ago."

Dr. Fossum sits on the edge of her armchair, leaning toward me. She asks, "Was leaving Cincinnati a good thing for you?"

It's a question that's never occurred to me. It radiates from memories I neglect. Even so, the memories haven't faded.

There I am, trying to pry myself from my father's grip as he drags me into the hospital. There I am, strapped down to a hospital bed flexing with all my might. There I am, pressed hard against the railing of my third-floor balcony. As these memories return to me, quiet becomes silence.

Of course, leaving was a good thing.

Wasn't it?

I think of my wife, my daughter, and the meaningful work I've done, all discovered and embraced since that time. But something is making me pause.

"My last two years in Cincinnati centered on bipolar disorder," I say. "I needed to get away from that. I needed a fresh start."

But it changed everything. Yes, I've gained so much since then, but how much did I lose?

Some paint has chipped off the wall behind Dr. Fossum's chair, and I stare at it as emotions long dormant begin to reemerge. I didn't come here to face my past. Why would I want to do that? So much fear, so much pain, and so many stories I don't know how to tell. I came here to find a way forward, but here I am, looking back.

Chapter 2

APRIL 11, 2004

CINCINNATI, OHIO

My typing punctuated the quiet. My parents and sister were in their bedrooms for the night. My girlfriend Kristin was in the guest room, adjoining the study where I worked. It was well past midnight. A term paper absorbed my complete focus. I scrolled up to its title, "Where Are the Unnaturally Wealthy in the Public International Human Rights Discourse? A Dangerous Omission as Seen through the Slave Trade."

The paper was for my favorite class in my international affairs major at Xavier University—Africa, Religion, and Human Rights—taught by Farid Esack, a visiting professor from South Africa. Farid was dear to my heart. He was provocative, direct, and challenging—all things I admired and aspired to be.

His understanding of international affairs diverged from the points of view I heard in my American professors' lectures. One day, Farid made our class squirm by observing that while the United States justified its invasion of Afghanistan, partly by a desire to liberate women—apparently one of our fundamental values—Afghanistan wasn't invading the US to impose its values on us.

"In Afghanistan, they revere elders and make great sacrifices to care for them in their homes until they die. In the United States, you send your elders to nursing homes and maybe visit them once a week," he said. A sly smile spread across his face. "So, why hasn't Afghanistan invaded the United States to liberate your elders?"

My classmates were silent, so he answered his own question. "Power."

Farid and I sometimes shared meals at the school café or in local restaurants. He paid every time, even when I ordered beer—something he refrained from as a devout Muslim. He believed that those with more wealth should pick up the bill. At that point, I hadn't told Farid about my own wealth and struggle to understand what it meant to be wealthy—the personal dilemma simmering beneath the carefully constructed academic argument in my term paper.

My research turned up a 1976 United Nations covenant on social and cultural rights, declaring that all people had the right to work for fair wages and provide a decent living for themselves and their families. The document focused almost entirely on workers—from safe and healthy working conditions to maternity leave, distribution of food, health care, and access to technology. But then, near the end, the rights of business owners were addressed: "Nothing in the present Covenant shall be interpreted as impairing the inherent right of all peoples to enjoy and utilize fully and freely their natural wealth and resources."

This sentence spawned my entire five-thousand-word term paper. I reasoned that if there was such a thing as *natural wealth,* then there must be *unnatural wealth,* which I defined as "wealth obtained by employing or using people (processors) to pursue and make profit (additives)."

If someone's wealth was bloated through profits or the labor of others, it wasn't natural; it was unnatural. The logical result was that the unnaturally wealthy didn't have the right to fully and freely enjoy and utilize such wealth. My examples of the unnaturally wealthy were the billionaire reality TV star Donald Trump and Captain Theophilus Conneau, a slave trader in Liberia during the early 1800s.

As my research and analysis wove together, my argument became more forceful and more powerful. A rush of adrenaline flooded me. I closed my eyes for a moment and felt my body pulse. My breath flowing through my nostrils. Heat radiating from my pores. The steady rhythm of my heart. My physicality aroused me.

Through the crack in the bifold door, I saw Kristin's silhouette under the covers. I rose from the desk chair, pushed the door open, and entered the guest room. I removed my clothes and slipped into bed beside her. My index finger drifted up her bare leg until it met her shorts, then curled just under the light fabric, and began sweeping around the circumference of her thigh. She stirred. She lay on her side facing away from me, but when I kissed her neck, she rolled onto her back and found my lips with hers. My intricate web of thoughts about economic injustice disappeared as I pulled her into me.

Afterward, I lay with her, our limbs pretzeled together. Her breath slowed, grew deep, and, when her hand slipped from mine, I left the bed and returned to the computer.

The screen lit up when I struck a key. My focus was back and all that remained to write was the conclusion.

"The loudest critique of the market economy," I wrote, "is that it has not done much to bridge the gap between the wealthy and the poor. If the goal of the market economy is to fairly exchange what we value, then we have the responsibility to ensure that the unnaturally wealthy do not impinge upon that fairness."

A light flashed through the window as I heard a car park in front of the house. I looked out the window and saw Patrick get out of my Dodge Neon.

Before he could knock, I opened the front door.

"Patrick, you're late."

The smell of alcohol hit me. His eyes were moist and narrow.

"Let's walk," I said as I took him by the arm and led him away from my parents' house.

When I met Patrick during my first year at Xavier, I had recently returned from a three-month internship in Kenya, his home country. Patrick had a magnetic pull on me. His dark skin broke up the monotony of a mostly white campus. I was invigorated by his jovial nature and his formal English peppered with Swahili. He connected me to a country that was thousands of miles away—one that had changed me—and that I was trying to change.

During my internship, I taught in a rural secondary school. I was eighteen years old and had always taken access to education for granted. The students I taught had to pay to attend school and sometimes didn't have enough money, so they were sent home until they paid.

When I learned this, I resolved to do something about it. So, when I got home, I started Ugali, an organization to pay the school fees of the students I taught during my internship. I dove into fundraising and began sending thousands of dollars back to Kenya. I had grand visions—Ugali would create a huge transfer of wealth, bring education to the masses, expand job opportunities, and eradicate poverty.

Then I met Patrick.

Before coming to America, Patrick had worked as a social worker for an organization that helped impoverished Kenyan students pay for their education—he knew how to target the use of funds to make strategic change. We began hanging out, and when summer came, off we went to Kenya.

With him by my side, I soon realized how little I knew and how naive I had been.

On our first trip, he tactfully helped me see the stratification of wealth in Kenya. There were many children in no need of help to get through school, including students Ugali had already sponsored. He introduced me to the concept of community-supported giving, where we partnered with women's groups that were familiar with local families and could direct donations where they had the most impact.

As he guided me along this process, I was humbled and learned how much I needed Patrick—someone who understood Kenya, who understood aspects of humanity I didn't, who could appreciate my confidence, and who could tolerate my ignorance.

During our days in Kenya, Patrick and I met with women's groups and talked with them about partnering with Ugali.

At night, we made memories.

If there was music in the air, we would find its source and dance the night away. We ate roasted goat at midnight. We laughed, played pool, and drank liters of warm Tusker, a Kenyan beer.

I was thousands of miles from home, often the only white person for miles. My gut hummed with anxiety and vulnerability. But I suppressed it, stifled my fears, and gave myself to the moment, to joy. I could—because I had Patrick.

In the two years after our first trip, we moved in together, built a community of friends, took road trips during school breaks, put on fundraisers for Ugali, gave presentations at schools about life in Kenya, and returned to Kenya in the summer. We became inseparable. I had never loved a friend with such intensity.

Now, here he was, drunk and sweating under the flickering streetlights, his eyes red and swollen. I held his arms, trying to steady him.

"What's wrong?"

"She's pregnant, Adam. She's giving birth." His lips quivered. His eyes squeezed shut. "There's a lot of blood."

I leaned in, shocked. "What?" I blurted. "Who are you talking about?"

The story spilled out.

A woman had called from Kenya. Patrick hadn't heard from her since we left the previous summer. I had met her in Kisumu through Patrick. She was around him a lot during our trip, and her presence made me uneasy because Patrick had a girlfriend back in Cincinnati.

Nine months later, he wept as he told me about the phone call. She was in the throes of an agonizing childbirth and called Patrick to ask for money. He was the father, she told him.

It was an odd time to make a call, but this didn't register with me at that moment. All I could see was my best friend crying, and it was wrenching. He was older. Stronger. He was my compass. I mimicked him in many ways, even switching my underwear choice from the boxers of my adolescence to Patrick's layering of briefs and athletic shorts under his pants.

"Patrick," I said with authority. "I'll talk to my parents tomorrow about getting some money out of my college account."

He looked up from the ground. His eyes were still pained, but some of the panic had dissolved. I put my arm around his shoulders as we walked back to the house. Once inside, I made up the sofa bed in the solarium and he collapsed into it. Before closing the pocket doors, I looked at him lying there, defeated, and resolved to help him in any way I could. Then I headed back upstairs to finish my paper.

Patrick's news made it hard to focus. I turned from the computer screen and looked out the window into the night. My thoughts drifted back to my first trip to Kenya, as they often did.

The Isiche family hosted me during my internship. They lived on a modest piece of land with an acre of crops, a cow, an outbuilding with a kitchen, a three-room house, and a second smaller house.

Joseph, the eldest child, in his final year of high school, lived in the smaller house—a traditional mud structure with a thatched roof. It had two slender rooms—one with a bed, the other with a chair at a small table, and a shelf holding his textbooks. When I arrived for my stay, Joseph insisted I sleep in his bed while he slept in the other room on a floor mat.

As I came to know life for the Isiche family and for my students, I filled my journal with insights about wealth and privilege and my plans to transfer wealth to those without it. But during the nights, lying under a mosquito net in Joseph's bed, my thoughts gave way to feelings.

Every night it began with Joseph's bed. I felt undeserving—of his bed, my plush sleeping bag, fancy backpack stuffed with clothes, thick stack of traveler's checks, and American passport. As I lay in a nest of Joseph's generosity, I felt an overwhelming impulse to give away everything I owned, to escape the loneliness of having wealth in a world where that was rare. And then, I felt terrible for not appreciating what I had.

Years later, sitting in front of my parents' computer, trying to finish my research paper, I struggled with those same feelings.

The line between my assignment and my life began to blur. Perhaps I wasn't unnaturally wealthy as I had defined it, but I knew I was wealthier than most people in the world and certainly most Kenyans I knew. Every time Patrick and I went to a bar and the bill came, every time my friends went to their jobs they needed to help pay for school, and every time I walked through the door of my large Victorian childhood home, I thought of my wealth. My next semester would be my last, and I still had over $100,000 in my college account. A pittance compared to Trump, but it felt like a fortune to me.

As the first glow of morning reached up into the sky, my concentration deepened, but something within me had shifted. The tight logic of my argument wasn't enough. For the unnaturally wealthy—and for me—to hold and use our wealth wisely, we needed something more than a rational argument to respect human rights. So, I left behind the rigid structure of a research paper and entered the realm of prayer.

> Unnatural wealth demands a daily regimen of gratitude. And while songs of praise may not find a choir, the unnaturally wealthy soul should sing daily, and that prayerful song might go something like this:

I'm so grateful.
I'm so grateful.
I'm so grateful.

But I'm so lonely, Lord.
I have a secret that nobody wants to hear,
I've received a gift that's hard to share.
Lord, help me not to grasp this gift too tightly,
But with open hands and fingers spread slightly.
So that this gratitude will seep through like sand,
Showering the people who reaped it from the land.
For they have given, and I've received
And honestly, Lord, I do believe
That this gratitude is theirs as much as mine,
That this is a cycle and not a line.
If I fail or grasp too tight,
Please smack my hand with loving spite.
Help me land my plane, Lord, so that I can see,
Why I've been feeling so awfully lonely.

I'm so grateful.
I'm so grateful.
I am, so grateful.

I clicked on save, printed the paper, and powered down
the computer.

Chapter 3

NOVEMBER 2, 2022
St. Paul, Minnesota

Nine people are seated in the circle of chairs at the bipolar, depression, and anxiety support group. The meeting is in a community center, about a ten-minute drive from my house. This is my second time coming. The facilitator, a volunteer who has depression, does a good job of ensuring everyone gets time to speak.

When it's my turn, I tell the group about my manic episode eighteen years ago during my senior year of college. I describe the fear, pain, anger, and pity I've felt since—when I remember it. I talk about how those feelings have overshadowed everything else about my college years. But I'm trying to change that. I'm trying to be kinder to my college self.

As I remember my college years now, in therapy and with the support group, I hold the hand of a twenty-one-year-old me.

Some people nod, others shift in their chairs. When I finish, the facilitator asks, "Do you still feel like you're the same person you were before you went manic?"

Everyone in the room takes a deep breath. For some, there is no before–they feel like they always struggled with some aspect of mental illness–but for many of us, there was. At that moment, I don't have an answer, but the question sticks.

The next week in therapy, I share the question with Dr. Fossum.

I tell her about my college self: long hair held back by a colorful woven band, chasing down a Frisbee on the campus green at night, hand thrust into the air in every class eager to contribute, lounging outside the international student center with friends from all over the world, putting on fundraisers for Ugali complete with speakers, food, and dancing. And there is more, so much more—so many memories I haven't allowed myself to remember.

Then I admit something I've pushed aside and tried to forget.

My voice is shaky but sure. "I loved myself."

I pause as my admission slices down years of forgetting. Forgetting I was so alive. So interesting. So filled with purpose.

With the admission comes sharp pain–familiar but dusty.

It's the pain I felt during those first two years after the manic episode, back when the memory of my old self was fresh—right at the tips of my outstretched hands—but so unreachable. He was gone, and I didn't know if he would ever come back, and I missed him so damn much.

Under the pressure of these memories, I begin to weep. The tears are new–eighteen years in and out of therapy with four therapists but few tears. This time is different. This time I'm not just solving an immediate problem. Quitting my job broke me wide open, and now I'm releasing all I've held inside.

"It was a long fall," I manage to say.

As the memories come back, my heart fills with admiration for the person I was before the manic episode. It's been a long time since I focused my attention on that version of myself. The searing grief of loss forced me to look away, remembering my college years only in snippets that didn't require a full reckoning. It is time for that to change.

When I get home from my session, I go straight to my wife's home office. Meredith hears me coming up the stairs.

"Hello, honey," she calls, chipper as ever.

I walk in and she must see heavy emotions on my face because she stands up and wraps her arms around me. She holds me tight, for as long as I need, waiting for the moment I squeeze her, then pull back.

I describe my session with Dr. Fossum. I tell Meredith how I'm trying to allow myself to love the person I was back before bipolar disorder, back before she met me. I tell her, in looking back, how interesting I seemed, how engaged, and how full of life.

Her face is soft, comforting. In a gentle voice, she says, "You're describing the person I know. The person I love. You are still all of those things."

Chapter 4

APRIL 11, 2004

CINCINNATI, OHIO

As the house filled with sunlight, euphoria surged through my body. The term paper was complete, and I was eager to turn it in and share these insights with Farid. I grabbed the paper from the printer, hurried downstairs, and slipped it into my backpack.

In the dining room, I found four envelopes on the heavy oak table. The Easter Bunny had visited while I was upstairs typing. Even though I was twenty-one and my sister Jessica had just turned eighteen, the tradition persisted, and at my request, this year there were envelopes for Kristin and Patrick as well. We would each get an Easter basket after deciphering the Easter Bunny's clues to their hiding places. Within that basket, there would be a clue to another and then another. Three baskets for each of us.

I picked up the envelope with my name on it. "Adam," was written in my father's distinctive scribble, setting off a cascade of memories. There was his handwriting on the letter I received from Santa Claus every Christmas morning. There was his handwriting on the brown paper lunch bag I grabbed from the refrigerator before school. There were the loving notes to the family left on the countertop in the early mornings before he disappeared for a week of depositions.

And there I was at the Isiches' home, reading and rereading his letters that had traveled across the Atlantic.

Al Gerhardstein had given so much to me and to this world, and he did this without a murmur of hope for reciprocity. How could I not have seen it? My father gave so much, yes, but he was as human as anyone else. Deep down in his soul, he would love to receive. How many Easter mornings had he watched his children scurry all over the house hunting for our baskets, following the clues he had written, and secretly wished that there was a basket for him? It was obvious what I had to do.

I found a piece of paper and a pen and wrote a clue to my father from the Easter Bunny. I had no candy or basket for him, but that wasn't important. What he needed was to see himself for who he was in the eyes of others—who he was in his son's eyes. Such a loving man. A giving man who had rarely received.

I wrote him a clue to help him see the depths of my appreciation for him. It led him to the bathroom mirror where he would see his face and understand how magnificent a father he was.

***

The morning air greeted me as I stepped out the front door and onto the porch. My eyes fluttered, and I took a deep breath as I pulled a pack of Marlboro Lights from my pocket. The first inhale erased the jitters of a sleepless night. With the cigarette between my fingers, I walked slowly along Wyatt Avenue, soaking up a beautiful dawn.

After passing a few houses, I came to a young maple, its leaves sparkling and coated with morning dew. Pale yellow-green, they were new to the world, beginning their life cycle while last year's leaves decayed. Their mesmerizing shimmering transported me to the realm of the eternal, where the current moment blends with all of history and the onward marching future.

The message came to me with force: the leaves were beginning anew, just as Christ rose from the grave on this Easter morning almost two thousand years ago. It was time for me to begin fresh as well. I was smoking my last cigarette. That chapter of my life was over. No more smoking. No more death.

The realization filled me with a sense of certainty—of destiny. This communion with God was new to me. Over the last couple of years, I had been on three spiritual retreats through Xavier's campus ministry, even helping lead the third one. Those retreats had fostered my confidence in my relationship with God and expanded my comfort with prayer.

As I looked at the tree shining in the sunlight, I knew my relationship with God had truly matured. We were in conversation now about things small and large. A real back-and-forth. A layer of loneliness that lived in my subconscious slipped away, and I tingled with sacred energy.

I let the cigarette fall from my fingers, stepped on it, and walked back toward the house.

My first Easter basket was hidden in the study's closet among my father's racquetball gear. After retrieving it, I turned back toward the hallway and saw my father in the bathroom looking into the mirror. I paused to witness the private moment I had orchestrated. Would he smile and bring his hands to his heart? Would he neatly fold the note and slip it into his pocket to save it forever? Would he turn and see me and enfold me in his arms?

He took off his glasses and set them on the bathroom sink. He brought his hands to his face. His olive skin twisted with raw emotion. And his entire body began to sob. I had seen him cry before but not like that. I wanted to run, but I couldn't move.

What did I write? What was causing him such pain? I had meant to give him a gift, like the many he had given me. My soul ached. What had I done? Then I understood: he had never received an actual Easter basket. He must have been so excited to get one when he saw my note and then I left him empty-handed. It made perfect sense: all the years of Easter "Bunny-ing" and never having the joy of the pursuit. I had given him a pathway to childhood, but like any child left unrewarded, my father was left with only his tears.

It was just my parents and me, gathered in the living room with Easter baskets still strewn about, and it was my turn to cry. Patrick and Kristin were back at Xavier. Jessica was at a friend's house.

It was still morning, and the sunlight hit our faces through the six-foot-tall easterly windows. I sat lower than my parents, in an antique chair pushed up against the wall, with the two of them across the room from me on the overstuffed couch.

I started with Patrick's dilemma.

"I need some money out of my college account," I said. "I need to help Patrick."

My father leaned in.

"Tell us more."

There was a lot my parents didn't know about Patrick. They knew he was poor. That he had found his way to the States through hard work, intelligence, and the goodwill of American Catholic priests who wanted him to succeed. He was in his early thirties, working toward his bachelor's, and spent most waking moments with his best friend—me.

My parents had helped pay for our travels to Kenya the two previous summers so we could continue building Ugali into a more sustainable organization. While there, I had stayed in the slums where Patrick had lived and traveled to his father's farmland on the border with Uganda. Patrick never had an easy life, but he was resilient and high-spirited, with a ready laugh and a beaming smile.

My parents knew all of that, but they didn't know about the pregnancy. Their image of Patrick was important to me, but in my desperate desire to help Patrick, I told them everything. All his secrets. All our secrets.

There was much to confess from the recent past.

There had been late nights. Many of them. Shooting pool, going to Cincinnati's African dance club, often driving home drunk with me steering and working the clutch while he shifted the gears from the passenger seat. I had been waking up for class just a few hours after going to bed, dry heaving as I stumbled toward campus.

Classes, for the first time, seemed less of a priority and more of a burden. I had dropped my Globalization course, unable to handle the fifteen credit hours I had breezed through each previous semester. I was considering dropping International Law as well.

Then there was our spring break road trip out East.

In one week, I slept with an old friend in Philadelphia and cuddled with one of my brother's roommates at Brown

University. Kristin and I weren't official yet, but I had no restraint; I was just bursting with lust. Patrick, left to fend for himself, grew so angry with me that he made me take him to the closest airport. I dropped him off at the curb and drove away. Unable to afford a ticket or find someone to pay for one, Patrick called me from a pay phone and said, "Adam, don't say a damn word; just pick me up."

We drove the fifteen hours from Rhode Island to Cincinnati in silence, a Jimmy Cliff CD playing on repeat. When I tried to break the silence at a Wendy's, Patrick wouldn't reciprocate.

In the five weeks since, we had patched up our friendship—partly out of necessity as we shared an apartment.

Two nights before Easter, we saved my sister's eighteenth birthday party. We borrowed my parents' van and dropped her and her friends off at a dance club downtown. But they wouldn't let in boys under twenty-one, so they all trudged back to my parents' van. Patrick and I knew what to do. We drove up to Mondiale, the African dance club where I had gotten my VIP card as a nineteen-year-old.

Confidently striding in with a gaggle of teenagers, we were greeted warmly and soon took over the dance floor, with the DJ shouting Jessica's name. I bought rounds of drinks until her teenage friends threw up in the bathroom. When the hefty bar tab came, I put it on my credit card. My treat.

Thirty-six hours later, I confessed my behavior to my parents, peeling back layers of emotion I had never felt before.

There was urgency. My best friend needed money, and I was in a position to help him, with just a little assistance from my parents. I needed them to loosen the purse strings.

My grandfather, Archie Gingold, a retired judge in St. Paul, Minnesota, owned some commercial properties and, through rents and a frugal lifestyle, saved a considerable sum—a portion of which he parceled out each year to his eight grandchildren for college education funds. Over the years, these gifts and their earned interest had compounded so that now, in my senior year of college, it was clear I would graduate without a dime of debt but with a hefty nest egg for whatever came next. The account was in my name, but it was under my father's control.

"Please," I begged. "I need some money to help Patrick."

My parents looked at each other. A silent message passed between them, and my mom said, "Your father and I are going to have to talk about how to handle this."

It wasn't the answer I hoped for, but it wasn't a no.

There was one more thing I had to mention. "I got my credit card bill. I'm going to need some money to pay that off as well."

My mom tensed. "You've already spent your semester's spending money?"

"Yes."

Silence.

My mom stiffened. "Give us your credit card."

"No," I snapped.

My mom didn't blink.

My mother is someone who never backs down. Mimi Gingold doesn't worry about the thickness of your skin. She understands people—all people—regardless of the languages they speak. In five minutes, she knows your life story.

My mother has been a teacher, librarian, and businesswoman. She has opened her home to refugees from Vietnam and Kosovo. She wore a green dress at her wedding. She loves the smell of skunk. Her sneezes are so dramatic they defy description.

What I'm trying to say is that my mother is unbreakable. Every time I've tried to break her, it's backfired.

Once, in my late teenage years, when she found out I was regularly smoking marijuana, she informed me I was going to need to get weekly drug tests to keep using their car. The next day, when I pulled up in front of the house with a rusted-out pickup truck bought with my life savings, I defiantly looked up at her standing on the porch. She shook her head, said we would talk when my father got home, turned her back, and walked into the house. The look of disappointment on her face was so sobering I haven't used drugs since.

My mom has opinions that she states as facts. Many people feel compelled to push back, challenge her, and try to get her to admit she might be wrong, or at least that there's another way to see the world.

Not me. I believe my mom is always right. Because I believe in my mother's infallibility, I am liberated. I feel no impulse to challenge her or change her. I believe in her rightness more than she does. Even when she admits a mistake, I see where she was coming from.

But right then, after pouring out my heart in the living room, I couldn't see where she was coming from. I didn't believe she was right. No, she was dead wrong.

"Your father and I are going to talk, but you will give us your credit card now."

"I'm not a child anymore," I said. "I'm twenty-one years old. I can handle my own finances."

"That's fine," she said, her voice steady. "We respect that. But since you don't have a source of income, we're not going to allow you to continue running up debt, thinking you can pay for it out of your college account. That money is for education."

Our eyes locked. I was desperate and angry, but she was determined.

The credit card was in my wallet. I removed it and held it in front of me. My parents watched as it fell from my hand and landed on the floor. I turned and walked out the door.

Chapter 5

NOVEMBER 7, 2022
St. Paul, Minnesota

When I open my email, I see a beautiful name in the "From" field. It's a name I haven't seen in many years, but one that has been on my mind a lot lately. "Farid Esack." My heart leaps. Therapy has brought me back to college, to the years he was last in my life. My favorite professor. My friend.

The subject line is simple: "Thinking of you." And the message is concise: "Warmly and learning. Warm regards, f."

Time seems to stop. There is nothing in the world but this email. Farid is thinking of me, and I am thinking of him. That is it, and it is more than enough beauty to brighten an entire month.

I draft a reply—a brief update about my life—and then I go deeper, into my illness, into my therapy. Before sending it, I reread it, and for some reason, I hesitate.

Is it too much?

Yes, I decide, so I edit out much of the depth and leave the surface. But he has been in my thoughts, so I at least tell him why.

"I was thinking of you because I am in a moment when bipolar disorder is at the forefront of my mind, which always makes me think about its onset at Xavier. I remain very grateful for your help at that time of crisis and for your friendship during my college years."

I send it off to him and his reply comes at once. With his typical bluntness, he apologizes and says that little I told him was new.

"In the time that we are living, there is stupidity, yes, but not a lack of information. I continue to love you despite–or because of—all. I have been going through piles of notes, letters, cards, files, articles, and mementos that I have gathered all my life and on many continents. I finished in the early morning hours, and three letters have emerged as the most precious for me to read and read and read over again so that I can learn from their ruthless and painful honesty. One is written by you."

I fall back into my chair and look up, away from my computer.

A memory forms, not a specific one but a construction— an honest construction, something real and true, a memory denied and buried, but now clawing its way out of the dark. There I am sitting at my college desk writing a letter, creating something of value, something to be treasured. And it was not a fluke. I remember it coming from a worthy heart, a deeply engaged mind, a person who cared, who gave it his all. I see a beautiful soul.

Hearing from Farid makes me think of Patrick. It's been many years since I've looked him up and checked on Ugali, so I open my web browser.

The Ugali website is beautiful. Patrick's smiling face graces the pages. The organization is still doing wonderful work in Kenya. On the IRS website, I see he's kept up with the nonprofit filings. My heart fills and my fingers hover over the keyboard as I think about our relationship since my manic episode.

Soon after my hospitalization, I moved out of our apartment. During the next few months, we hung out a couple times, but then we drifted apart. Our communication was limited to the business of handing over control of Ugali and the occasional "I'm thinking of you" email when events in Kenya made international headlines. Eighteen years of distance after two years of brotherhood.

At first, I was incapable of maintaining relationships. My manic episode was followed by a deep depression that walled me off from everyone. But, as I got better and grew more capable of connecting with others, I didn't rekindle my friendship with Patrick.

For many years, I justified my silence by clinging to memories of his dishonesty and a few personal matters he had withheld from me, as if I was entitled to know everything—*everything*—about his life.

But it wasn't just Patrick. I walked away from every friend, every professor, and every mentor I had made in college. All except Kristin, and even that relationship eventually ended. In my muddled mind and traumatized soul, that manic episode at the end of senior year got conflated with every aspect of my college experience. The mere thought of contacting my college friends triggered flashbacks, and only now, eighteen years later, am I finding the emotional strength to see the memories of my mania with kindness rather than fear.

But my silence has come at a cost. Patrick's absence from my life has been an open wound that I know, deep down, will never heal without him. As I look at his face on my computer screen, an intense longing sweeps over me.

Should I write? Call? For days I mull this over. I try to find the courage to reach out and connect. *But what will I say? What could I possibly say?*

In the end, I donate. I send a $250 check and pray he responds. A couple weeks later, a stock thank-you card arrives. "Thanking you for your kindness…" it says on the front. I open it. "…and thanking God for you." Signed, "Patrick."

Walking to Dr. Fossum's office, I think of Patrick's card.

"I got a thank-you card from Patrick," I say toward the end of our session.

A long pause.

"I wrote him back."

I look down and take a moment to collect myself. "If I'd written him a letter last year or any time before, I would have said, 'I'm sorry,' but I didn't say that."

My body is tense from head to toe. And then it all escapes.

"I just said 'I miss you.'"

Dr. Fossum hands me a tissue. I wipe my eyes over and over again. My nose starts to run, and I mop up the snot. It's a long time before I can speak again.

She watches me from the edge of her chair, her posture somehow conveying empathy. Our eyes finally meet.

"We were a force." I bring my fists together in front of my body. "Like this. And we both contributed to that force." I drop one of my fists on the couch. "And then I disappeared."

APRIL 12–13, 2004
CINCINNATI, OHIO

Money. I needed money. It was all I could think about as I drove around town. When I passed Betta's, an Italian restaurant on a nearby corner, only a few blocks from campus and frequented by many students and professors, an idea formed.

I would get a job as a server and, as I moved between the tables, I would overhear the conversations of professors and students. After work, I would write amusing columns about what I heard for the *Newswire*, our campus newspaper. I would get paid by the restaurant and paid for the column. The *Newswire* would love the idea; I was sure. And what about the articles I already wrote? They brought so much depth to the paper, and they had cost me dearly, but I wasn't paid a dime.

Over the previous six months, they had published four opinion pieces I authored. I wrote one piece about how the United States was exploiting the oil resources of Equatorial Guinea. I wrote another about the absurdity of a country where President Bush talked about "defending the sanctity of marriage" in the same month that Britney Spears got married in a baseball cap veil only to have her marriage annulled three days later—a series of events her record company called "a joke gone too far."

Two months before Easter, I wrote an article entitled "Our Whiteness" about the oppressive history of white American men. That article generated a backlash. Some students let me know to my face they didn't agree, and one published a rebuttal defending the many just and praiseworthy white men my article didn't recognize.

I responded with an article called, "My Letter to the Readership." In it, I disclosed my pathway to my opinions—my travels to Africa, as well as the details of a conversation with a Black friend about how she carried the weight of her ancestors' sacrifices and suffering when she went to class every day. I named her and shared what she had told me in private, without thinking about how she might feel about that exchange being made public. All I considered was how learning her story made me realize how little responsibility I felt for my ancestors' actions. She didn't appreciate having our personal discussion published, and our friendship was fractured.

Sharing my opinions in the *Newswire* cost me a friend, and I had earned nothing. It was time to get what I was due. Those articles were probably worth hundreds with the controversy they had caused.

The *Newswire* offices were right in the heart of campus in a hundred-year-old brick house. I found the editor-in-chief on the second floor, seated at his desk, with a computer screen lighting his face. I stayed standing as I asked to be paid for my articles. He said no—they didn't pay for voluntary submissions. He equated my articles with all the others. I was in disbelief.

"This is bullshit!" I yelled.

The injustice of it filled the room, and I called him out. His eyes were wide as I harangued him, making my case for payment. The other newspaper staff in the room stared, transfixed, and those working on the floor below crept up the stairs to see what was going on. Everyone was quiet and stunned, but I was on a roll. I spoke with furor and purpose. Words flowed from me effortlessly. Eventually, the editor broke in with a shaky voice and said, "Look, we can give you ten dollars for each op-ed, but I can't give it to you now."

Ten dollars, I thought, *that's crazy. My submissions were worth ten times that.*

"Fine," I said. It was a start.

The bodies around me were tense, but I was relaxed, clear on my mission, and clear on my needs.

With forty dollars secured, I pitched him my idea to write a weekly column about being a waiter at Betta's serving students and faculty. I hadn't applied for the serving job yet, nor would I without the promise of the column.

He seemed uneasy. Instead of looking me in the eyes, he kept glancing at his colleagues.

"Well, what do you think?" I asked.

"Umm…" He paused. I stared at him, willing him to accept, I knew the column would be a gift to the paper. "We don't currently need any more regular contributors."

Disgusted, I snarled at him and stalked down the stairs and out of the building.

The next morning, I slipped my key into the lock of my parents' front door.

It had been another sleepless night, but I had clarity now and a message to deliver. When I turned on the bedroom light, their heads jerked toward the door, eyes blinking in the sudden brightness.

My dad put on his glasses. "What are you doing here Adam?"

"I brought you coffee. And I have a letter to read." It was a heartfelt letter that I had finished an hour earlier at 4:15 a.m.

They stared as I began. "Thank you so much for raising me."

Words of love, independence, and invitation tumbled forth.

"I deeply respect the both of you. I look forward to developing an adult relationship with you. I know that I am still your child, but I ask you to know that I am no longer a child."

I asked for my credit card back and then, reflecting on our Easter morning talk, I continued. "The reason I fell apart this weekend is that my life is so amazing, and I knew that you didn't quite know how amazing it is, and I wanted you to know. But I have found peace with the fact that you will never know, nor will anybody else. I am the only person in this world who will ever know how amazing a gift I was given the day I was born."

I concluded the letter. "I am ready to start taking care of myself. Thank you for getting me to this point. I couldn't have done it without you."

The room was still. They were motionless but now fully awake.

"Adam," said my mom, in a measured voice. "Promise us that you'll call a psychologist."

They hadn't even sipped the coffee I made for them.

"Mom, I don't need your help."

I walked out of their bedroom.

Later that day, I realized my stomach was empty and had been for quite a while. *When was the last time I ate?* There was a Subway at a nearby gas station.

"I'll have a foot-long turkey sub," I told the sandwich-maker.

He loaded on the cheese, turkey, lettuce, tomato, onion, and cucumber, squirted on a little bit of mayo, then sprinkled some oregano, salt, and pepper. With each topping, my hunger grew. With each movement, I studied the precise placement of the veggies, the imprecise line of mayo, the fold of the bread, and the slice through the middle, the wrapping. Every millimeter of that sandwich was internalized as if I had already eaten it.

As I drove the backstreets toward my apartment with the sandwich in the passenger seat, one song played on a loop from my CD player—Cindy Morgan's "How Could I Ask for More."

A month earlier, I had awoken to the song on the radio and chose to play it at the Encounter Retreat, the spiritual retreat I helped lead for Xavier's campus ministry. I gave a thirty-minute testimonial about my relationship with my mother and my growing relationship with God. At the end of the testimonial, I played the Cindy Morgan song, which exuded peace and gratitude.

Now, a month later, as I drove the streets of Cincinnati, I mouthed the words, and Cindy's sweet voice penetrated my soul. Accompanied by only a piano, every word came out of the speakers like a prayer, bringing sustenance and a sense of order. It reminded me of the many blessings in my life, and there were so many blessings—so so so many blessings.

By the end of the song, as I mouthed the final words every three minutes, I cried, over and over again, on loop.

Suddenly, Cindy's voice receded and a new one hit me.

It was God. Clear—as if God was a passenger in my car.

The message wasn't coded or vague; it was direct and forceful. God told me that if my older brother didn't propose to his girlfriend, she might hurt herself or even take her life. This truth had never occurred to me, but God's message was unequivocal, and it made perfect sense.

Ben and Katy had been dating for four years. They met as counselors at a summer camp. After that summer, they both started college—Ben at Skidmore, in upstate New York, and Katy at Brown, in Providence, Rhode Island. For two years, they kept their relationship alive by spending weekends and breaks together, despite the two-hundred-mile distance between their schools.

Then Ben transferred to Brown. Two years later, they were on the cusp of another major transition. They were about to graduate and go out into the working world. Thanks to God, it was obvious to me that Katy needed to know that Ben would always be there for her. She needed certainty. She couldn't go through another transition without a full, lifelong commitment. Ben had to give that to her. It was a matter of life and death.

I raced to my apartment, jumped out of my car, bolted up the steps, dropped the sandwich on our kitchen table, dashed into my room, flipped through my phone list, picked up my landline, and called Ben.

When he came to the phone, summoned by his roommate, I told him that he had to propose to Katy.

"Please," I told him. "Trust me…she is going to hurt herself if you don't."

Chapter 7

DECEMBER 6, 2022
St. Paul, Minnesota

My phone lights up on the counter. It's a text from our former next-door neighbor, Teresa.

"I wanted to share part of Sara's letter to Santa… 💔"

Sara is Phoenix's best friend, and I enlarge the picture of her Santa letter. One of the items on her wish list is for "Phoenix to come back." I feel like I've been punched in the gut.

Since I left Cincinnati sixteen years ago, I've moved three more times. This latest one has been the hardest by far. We moved to St. Paul, Minnesota, six months ago. Oddly enough, the city we came from was Cincinnati.

When I left Cincinnati as a twenty-three-year-old, I embraced a new life and thought I would never go back. But seven years later, after I was married to Meredith, life surprised me when I accepted my father's job offer to practice law with him in Cincinnati. Seven years away had changed me, and it had changed the city. It felt more like moving to a brand-new city than a homecoming.

Once there, I tried to keep my distance from the places where my ghosts lived—Xavier's campus, Good Samaritan Hospital, and my old apartment building in Clifton. And that wasn't too hard. There was plenty of city left to fall in love with, which we slowly did.

Meredith got a great job; I learned to be a lawyer; and Phoenix was born. We built a comfortable life for her within a loving circle of friends and my parents. After six years, I burned out as an attorney, and I got trained as a Montessori teacher for young children. I fell in love with the profession as I worked part-time at Phoenix's school.

But from the time we arrived in Cincinnati, Meredith and I talked about moving to Minnesota, where Phoenix had cousins and where Meredith was from. Cincinnati had never been in our plans, and we never made new ones, even after living there for nine years. With Phoenix finishing kindergarten, and my Montessori training ending, we figured it was a natural time to finally move to Minnesota.

We arrived in St. Paul in June 2022. It was only then that I realized how attached I had become to Cincinnati. And I didn't anticipate how hard the move would be for Phoenix. Leaving Sara broke my little girl's heart.

Sara was almost another daughter to us. She was four years older than Phoenix—ten and six, respectively, when we moved—but they could play from first light to dessert without a moment of discontent. We took her everywhere we went—to the pool, the Cincinnati Zoo, shopping for art supplies, the neighborhood library, Broadway shows at the Aronoff, and we even took her camping. None of us wanted to leave her, not just Phoenix. But we did.

And now I must live with it.

When I tell Dr. Fossum about Sara's wish list, I choke up, and Dr. Fossum nudges the tissues toward me.

I tell Dr. Fossum about our Cincinnati street, our neighbors, our wonderful friends, the nearby parks, our simple existence, and Phoenix's best friend. Every day I think of the life we left behind in Cincinnati and can't help but compare it to the life we're just beginning in St. Paul.

Dr. Fossum, back on the edge of her armchair, says, "It sounds like you need to grieve this loss."

I tense. She's struck a nerve. I've never been good at grieving. I've kept this shortcoming to myself and never asked for help. Until now.

"How do I do that?" I ask.

"Well, you have to honor what you've lost."

Afterward, walking home on sidewalks lined with snow-banks, I think of all the losses I've endured in my life, and I think of the last time I really grieved any.

It was my Nonna's death when I was eighteen. She was the embodiment of warmth. Her hugs, her smiles, and her food all nourished me. When she died, I wept. I remembered her beauty. At her funeral, I sang and participated in all the Catholic rituals even though they weren't familiar to me. I spoke about her. I thought about her often with love. I grieved her death with all my heart. Now, her death seems like an uncomplicated loss, the grief straightforward.

Somewhere between Dr. Fossum's office and our St. Paul home, I realize I've never grieved what I lost to my manic episode and diagnosis with bipolar disorder—something that's stunted my grief ever since. The loss was so big and unfathomable that I didn't realize I needed to grieve it or how to do so.

Instead of honoring my life before bipolar disorder, I clawed my way back to functionality and then pushed the past away. I didn't consciously repress or hide it, but I didn't recognize it either.

I bumbled along with a repository of loss ungrieved, and that became my pattern, loss after loss.

But now, this is changing—witness all those tears in Dr. Fossum's office. I'm finally learning how to grieve. And nothing could be more beautiful or devastating.

Chapter 8

APRIL 13, 2004
CINCINNATI, OHIO

My memories of what happened between Kristin and me during my manic episode are snapshots held together by a thread. Soon after Easter, our relationship frayed, we argued, and conflict grew. I don't remember the trigger or the content of our dispute—if there even was a cogent subject matter—but I remember trying to address it, understand it, and fix it. There is a progression and a manic logic to what I did, but the memories themselves are short—sharp but brief.

The chain pharmacy was open twenty-four hours. Inside, I saw a large bin of cheap inflated balls that kids love to play with. Immediately, I understood that it was time to put the ball in her court. I grabbed a blue one.

Farid and I walked toward campus. He was wearing a big grin, and I was carrying my blue ball. I headed to Kristin's apartment. He walked me to the front of her building, and we parted ways.

I slipped into the building and rushed up the stairs. With a flourish, I swung open the door of the apartment.

Amanda, Kristin's roommate, appeared startled as she watched me stroll through the living room holding the blue ball. Kristin wasn't there. I stepped into her bedroom and placed the ball on her bed. It was in her court now.

Her phone was on her desk, and I slipped it into my pocket. I laughed to myself as I walked past Amanda and out of their apartment.

Kristin's phone rang. "Hello?"

"Adam, why the hell did you steal my phone?"

"If you're not going to listen to me," I said, "then you're not going to listen to anyone."

"Bring my phone back right now. I need my phone."

Why didn't she understand? Why wouldn't she listen? It was so clear. If only she would let me explain.

"Where are you?" She demanded. "I will come and get it if I have to."

It was too much. Kristin. My parents. My brother. Three sleepless nights. There was no way I could make it to class that day. I intercepted Farid as he was rushing toward the side entrance of the academic building.

"Farid," I said, "I can't make it to class today. I'm too tired. Will you—"

He cut me off. "Adam. Okay. I don't have time. I'm late."

And he disappeared through the door.

What had I done? The pain was crushing, drawing tears. I had lost a friend.

I trudged across campus, disheartened, and, after being awake for seventy-six hours, utterly exhausted. My bed beckoned me. But the thought of walking from campus to my apartment, a mere two blocks, was overwhelming. The slight incline ahead of me looked like a mountain. Just then, the campus shuttle pulled to the curb. God had provided.

It was the middle of the afternoon, not a busy time, so I had the shuttle to myself, and I sat near the front to speak with the driver. In just two blocks, I learned that the shuttle service was going to be thinned and the driver was going to lose his job. Unbelievable.

I thought of all the other people who rode the shuttle, many more dependent than me—and the university was going to reduce the shuttle hours and fire someone who needed a job? The injustice was here, now. My sleep could wait. Despite my exhaustion, I knew I had to do something.

"I will write to Father Graham," I told the driver, "And ask him not to cancel the shuttle."

I got off the shuttle, ran up to my room, and started composing a letter to Father Graham, the university president.

"I write to you today on behalf of myself and God," the letter began. I thanked him for his leadership of the university where my relationship with God had developed. "I was raised as a Unitarian Universalist," I wrote. "We do not mention the G word or the JC word unless they are carefully premised and explained. Like most people, I greatly fear those things which I do not understand. Like most people, I also greatly admire those things which I do not understand."

Then I credited him with my choice to attend Xavier and explained that: "I have had to pull all my strength together to graduate. I needed a university that would kick my ass, and that is exactly what Xavier has done to me. It has been a real challenge, but I have met it."

I then pivoted to the task at hand: "I know I will be getting a diploma, but it has been very hard for me to earn that diploma, so I feel that I deserve a little something special. I have heard a rumor that you are thinking of canceling the daytime shuttle next year. Well, that shuttle and its kind driver have really helped me get home on those days when my load was so heavy that I simply couldn't walk. I needed that shuttle's help to carry my load. I have made some friends here who I will be leaving behind, and I imagine that their loads will only get heavier when I leave. Please don't cancel the shuttle."

There was one last thing he needed to know. He needed to see a glimpse of my loneliness. So I wrote, "It is hard being a white, middle-class, Unitarian Universalist, public school kid—who grew up in a diverse neighborhood, who had extremely liberal parents and who has traveled to Europe and Africa—when you feel surrounded by white, conservative, suburban, private school kids who you suspect just don't understand you, and you are doing everything you can to share yourself with them."

I printed the letter and walked down to the Commons Apartments, where Father Graham lived among the students. I entered the building, took the elevator to the top floor, and slid the note under his door.

Kristin's apartment was in the same building as Father Graham's, just downstairs, and so I headed her way.

Her apartment door was locked. For the first time, they had locked their door. I knocked.

"Go away, Adam." It was Amanda's voice.

"Please let me in. I need to talk with Kristin."

Silence.

I banged on the door. "Let me in!"

Silence.

I turned my back to the door, leaned against it, and slipped down onto the floor. Words streamed out of my mouth.

I lay down, announcing that I was lying down and wasn't going anywhere. I would wait for all eternity if I had to. Only next to her could I sleep, and if that hallway was as close as I could get, then that was where I would sleep.

Suddenly, the full history of our relationship raced through my mind as I pictured her on the other side of that door. The fact that we were together was a dream fulfilled.

It began two years earlier, in Kaufman Hall, when I moved into the dorms in January after transferring to Xavier from the University of Cincinnati. My mom and I were unloading my things from the elevator when two female students walked out of the girls' wing. I looked up, and they were smiling.

That was the first time I laid eyes on Kristin. She was gorgeous—tall, with long wavy brown hair, and a cute face with big wondrous brown eyes. We introduced ourselves, smiled, and then she disappeared into the stairwell. I watched her walk away and thought, *Yes, I want that girl.* I didn't know then that once inside the stairwell, Kristin turned to her friend and said, "He's mine!"

Despite our instant attraction, it would take two years for us to act upon it.

At the time, I wore my hair long and often sported a wide-brimmed soft leather hat. I also had a Turkish tea set, and Kristin loved my tea. She would come to my dorm room, and we would chat as my coffeemaker dripped hot water onto chamomile tea bags. As the new guy moving into the dorms midyear, I appreciated those moments deeply. What I didn't know then was that those moments were of great comfort to her as well.

Years later, when I first visited her childhood home, her grandmother sat me down at the kitchen table and made me a cup of tea. It was a ritual from Kristin's youth that I had unknowingly re-created at college.

Our friendship grew in a staggered fashion, with intense periods of connection followed by long lulls. Sometimes we teetered on the edge of romance but always stopped short. There was the night when her roommate was out of town and we danced in her dorm room late into the night to songs too slow for just friends, our bodies close but never closing the final distance.

Then there was the summer night in Cleveland, her hometown, where I had traveled with my dad to help him with a case. After the workday, I gave Kristin a call and then picked her up. We explored the city, laughing and leaning into our youth.

When I dropped her off, she told me to wait. She ran into her house and came back with an armful of blankets. We reclined the backseat of my parents' van and spent the night in her driveway, giggling, spooning, barely sleeping, but the sexual tension held. And then it was senior year, and the tension broke. We found ourselves in each other's arms and fell into each other with the passion of an instant attraction restrained for two years.

"I need to talk to Kristin!" I cried through the door. She had to understand. She had to listen. I needed to wrap my arms around her. The distance between us was killing me.

They kept telling me to leave. I banged my head against the door. Then a thought, and I was gone.

Chapter 9

DECEMBER 13, 2022

St. Paul, Minnesota

Here I am, married to Meredith for twelve years, the great love of my life—and thinking about Kristin.

I still feel guilty all these years since we broke up. I'm the one who left, and I wasn't always kind.

I feel no longing, no long simmering desire—just an emptiness and a big question mark in my soul in the place where my love for her once resided.

The internet tells me she's had interesting jobs, she's run a marathon, she's gotten married. She wore a happy smile in many of the pictures I found. But I want to know more than I can find online.

I talk to Meredith and Dr. Fossum about my thoughts of Kristin and my urge to reconnect with her.

Dr. Fossum suggests a letter.

"You are good with words," she says.

So, I write.

I tell Kristin that bipolar disorder has returned to the forefront of my mind. I tell her I've reconnected with Patrick, figuring that she, of all people, will understand what that means to me. I tell her I looked her up online and am glad she has a life of substance and community. I tell her I'm writing this book.

But I don't say what I've wanted to say for so many years: *Thank you, thank you for loving me even when I didn't love myself.*

She could have left. She could have turned her back on me—but she didn't.

As I write my letter, for the first time it occurs to me that maybe she didn't leave, not because she wanted to help or heal me, but because even during those early years of my illness, when I was first so manic and then so severely depressed, I was worthy of love. I was lovable. And then I see what I really want to say, what I really want her to know: that I still value her, and I remember.

Chapter 10

APRIL 13–14, 2004

CINCINNATI, OHIO

One night. Two nights. Three nights. On the fourth, I laid down to sleep, but my mind was raging. Impulses, insights, urges to action.

I needed help to calm down.

My friend Shangwe, from Tanzania, was staying over at our apartment. She was a good friend, unpretentious and kind, with a disarming giggle that brought sure smiles. Yes, her calm energy could help.

She was sleeping in Patrick's room. I woke them up.

"Shangwe, I'm having trouble sleeping." She raised her head from her pillow. "Could you snuggle me? I think it might help."

There was a moment of silence as she sat up and blinked the sleep out of her eyes. She focused her gentle gaze on me, filled with compassion and a dash of something else—something I hadn't seen before. *Was it wariness? No, it couldn't be.*

"I can do that," she said.

In my room, we crawled into my single bed together. I wrapped my arms around her, spooning her, and felt her warm body press up against mine. My lungs filled with a deep breath, and, with the exhalation, my body sank into the mattress.

My mind cleared for a moment, and it was just Shangwe and me. Our bodies. The bed. The quiet in the middle of the night. Yes, there it was, calm. Sleep was nearby.

My body veered toward sleep, but on the way there, it brushed past Shangwe's rear. Her ample bottom nestled in my crotch. Her coarse hair rubbed against my cheek. Her inviting scent filled me.

My heart quickened. My mind was foggy, but my body became fully aroused. My hands began to wander, my hips gyrated.

Shangwe pulled away, breaking my rhythm, and triggering a new thought. My mind focused into a sharp clarity. *What about Kristin? What was I doing? I had a girlfriend.*

"Shangwe, I think you should leave."

She got up and walked to the foot of the bed, where she paused and looked at me with those compassionate eyes tinged with that touch of something new. Then she went into Patrick's room and closed the door.

God needed something from me. I couldn't sleep. I had to prove to God that I believed. I would give God my breath. It would be my sacrifice.

I rolled onto my chest, shoved my body upward into a push-up position, and held myself tight.

I took deep breaths, chest heaving, ready to prove to God that I believed. On the tenth breath, I sucked in as much air as possible and held it. I felt strong, as strong as I ever had. I knew I was capable of denying myself oxygen to the point of death.

The clock ticked. My heart beat. My toes began to tingle. The tingling spread throughout my whole body. My head began to feel light, and my lungs cried out for a release, but I held strong. I had flirted with God long enough; it was time to commit. I was putting myself in God's hands. Would I live? Would I die? It was up to God. There was no greater way to prove my belief to God and to me.

I wanted to pass out and awaken in the glory of God's love. Alive or dead. I wanted to let go of the burdens weighing me down. I wanted to be cleansed. I wanted to be loved.

I fought against my breath, which desperately wanted release from my lungs until my whole body burned for air. At the pinnacle of my struggle, I collapsed onto my squeaky bed and my breath released with a whoosh. I bounced up and down, and felt the air rush back into my lungs.

My heart raced, and my body sparkled. For the first time in days, my mind was completely calm.

Clear.

Empty.

Then it came to me: God loved me. God didn't want me to stop breathing, God wanted me to live!

This beautiful realization filled my eyes with tears. This was foolishness, all of it. I needed to cleanse myself of it and be one with God.

I went into the bathroom and turned on the shower as hot as it would go. Steam filled the bathroom as I went into Patrick's room and woke him up. Shangwe also stirred.

"Patrick, I'm going to baptize myself." He got out of bed and looked at me through sleepy eyes. "Will you bless my towel?"

He took my towel from me, looked me up and down, and handed it back. He stood there watching me as I left his room.

In the bathroom medicine cabinet, I found a new bar of soap. I unwrapped it and stepped into the shower and scrubbed every inch of my body. As the soap ran down my face, I left my eyes open to cleanse my vision. I covered my hands with a thick film of soap, rubbed them together, and then stuck them into my ears and mouth to cleanse my hearing and speech.

Half an hour later, I emerged fresh. I was blessed.

Refreshed, I slid open our apartment window, lit a cigarette, and soaked in the night. The only sound was the cool wind rustling the early spring leaves. The birds were quiet, the crickets were quiet, and the cars were quiet, at rest in their garages.

Everything was calm, except my mind.

I asked and answered questions faster than any game show, any lightning round, or any human had ever done before.

I asked myself, "What am I going to do with my life?"

And I answered, "I'm going to law school and will become a lawyer, like my father and grandfather."

Just like that—I knew, I felt it—my grandfather, Judge Archie Gingold, died. It hit me hard.

For the first time, I saw what should have been so clear—how had I missed it? He wanted a lawyer in the family and had paid for his grandchildren's education, secretly hoping someone would follow in his footsteps. Now, I would.

My decision had been instantaneously transmitted into his consciousness. I saw it happen. He was asleep in St. Paul, Minnesota. His eyes closed, a faint smile crept across his face, and then life left his body. Finally, he could rest in peace. I checked the clock. Time of death: 2:15 a.m.

I was terrified. If I had only known what I was capable of, I would have been more careful with my thoughts. But it was too late.

I knew my phone would ring in the morning once my grandfather was discovered, and the devastating news moved through our close-knit family. I wrote Patrick a letter.

"I believe in people," I told him. "If the phone rings, Patrick, it's not because of God; it's because of me. It's because I had the courage to respond to God's call, even though I wasn't sure if I was doing the right thing."

The truth spilled forth as I told Patrick that he had introduced me to God. "You were my John the Baptist." And I had seen so much compassion in him that I tried to mimic him.

"This was not conscious," I wrote. "I was merely so in love with you that I forgot about myself."

I asked that, if the phone rang, he would take me to my parents' house and get me inside the door, "for I will not be able to walk on my own."

In the postscript, I asked if he thought it was a good idea for me to write my grandfather's eulogy with my cousin Andy.

———

The first thing I wanted Kristin to know when she woke up was that I loved her. The sun was rising, its light dancing across the sky and warming my face as I leaned out the living room window, smoking another cigarette. I headed for the door, but Patrick stopped me. He had just come out of his room moments ago. The letter was taped to his bedroom door, but the phone call hadn't come.

"Where are you going?" he asked.

"To get Kristin coffee at Starbucks."

"I'll drive you," he offered.

What a friend!

Thirty minutes later, he dropped me off at her student apartment building. It required a card to enter, so I waited by the back door for a resident to come out so I could slip in. It was only 7:00 a.m., so the wait was long. When the door finally opened, I charged in and ran up the stairs.

Quietly, I opened the door to her apartment, relieved it was unlocked, careful not to wake her roommates. I slipped into her bedroom and found her still asleep, her lovely face on her pillow.

Kneeling next to her bed, my mind raced through our two years of friendship and our recent commitment. I leaned in and kissed her nose. She opened her eyes and saw my face just inches away.

"I brought you coffee," I said with a smile.

She looked so peaceful, snuggled up in her blanket. I just wanted to crawl in and put my arms around her.

"I also figured out why we're fighting. It's because of our grandparents. You see—"

"Adam, it's early," she interrupted, "What are you talking about? Please leave."

Since writing the letter to Patrick, I had been mulling it over, trying to figure out why there was a rift between us—why I had taken her phone, why she had yelled at me, and why she had locked me out of her apartment. When it finally came to me, I wrote it all out.

"Activism and spirituality are two different responses to the emotion of compassion. Kristin and Adam, as people, experience compassion; what differentiates them is how they respond to their compassion."

In the "argument" section of the paper, I showed how I was most influenced by my mother, who was most influenced by her father, who responded to compassion with action. I showed how Kristin was most heavily influenced by her grandmother, who responded to compassion with concern. The argument had a parallel structure, comparing our family backgrounds. As I wrote, I saw how our dilemma had an obvious similarity to the conflict between Muslims and Christians. I made this explicit in the conclusion.

"It would seem that frustration, anger, and violence will continue between Muslims and Christians as long as they do not regularly visit each other's places of worship and learn how to see God through more than just one prophet."

After that long night and its many epiphanies, Kristin and I were face to face. I had figured it all out. The explanation was on paper, in my hand, but I needed to explain it to her. She needed to see the truth. But she was telling me to leave. *No, no, no!*

She sat up in bed. "Adam. Go!"

My head was throbbing. This was the moment. If she would only just listen. She was distracted and confused. She needed clarity and focus.

I pushed her back down into the bed by her shoulders and held her down.

"Don't you see? We are fighting because of our grandparents!"

"Adam!" She screamed. Footsteps started coming toward the door.

Chapter 11

JANUARY 1, 2023
St. Paul, Minnesota

It's New Year's Day. Phoenix is downstairs decorating gingerbread houses. Meredith is out skiing on the deep snow blanketing Minnesota.

I stand in our bedroom looking out the window at the white landscape, holding my phone in my right hand. The screen is lit up, and Patrick is pulled up in my contacts. I lift the phone and my finger hovers over his phone number. My eyes drift back up and out the window.

What will I say? How will he react? Will he even answer?

I search my memory for any substantive conversation we've had since I sank into depression eighteen years ago. Nothing memorable. It is hard to believe.

Tentatively, I touch the phone and it begins to ring.

He answers.

"Hello, Patrick, this is Adam."

Patrick gasps. "Adam!"

And then he begins to talk, and I settle in to listen. He speaks about his life over the past eighteen years. He tells me he's been a father to the child he learned of that Easter Eve. He's gotten married. His brother came to the States to study and then work.

Then Patrick tells me about going to prison. Drunk, he

fell asleep at the wheel, and another person was hurt in the crash. During the legal proceedings, he thought of reaching out to my father or me, but he chose not to. I feel a blow to my gut as a wave of guilt hits me. But he tells me his time in prison was meaningful. He built a community, taught classes, and was released after less than two years. When he got out, he quit drinking and spent more time with the most important people in his life. Throughout it all, he kept Ugali alive.

His voice is so familiar, so comforting, it's like listening to music. The tempo, the inflection, the laughter, the sorrow: it's the soundtrack of my college years.

When there is a lull, I speak and tell him the story of my disappearance. How my diagnosis traumatized me. How it was like a death, and I didn't know how to grieve. I tell him I'm not in touch with anyone from college. I tell him I'm in therapy, and I'm starting to see those years with different eyes—more compassionate eyes. I'm trying to embrace those memories, and that's what brought me to call. Because I miss him, and I have for many years.

"I'm glad you said that, Adam," Patrick says. "Friendship is strong to me. It can withstand many challenges. I didn't know much about bipolar disorder back then. I read some about it. But that didn't matter to me. You are my friend and that is all that matters. I waited one day, then two, then three. I waited for you, but you never came back." His voice slumps. "That was very hard."

The conversation continues. We reminisce. We hold our history together. After an hour, we begin our goodbyes and wonder where our relationship will go from here. We leave it open as we hang up.

Throughout the conversation, I paced back and forth

in my bedroom. But now I stop and return to the window to look out at the snow.

He waited for me, and I never came back.

It echoes in my head.

He could have reached out to me, and perhaps he did. It has been so long I can't be sure, but I was the one who went into hiding, and I was the one who never came out. Until today.

The stories he told from his last eighteen years scroll through my mind, but in them, I see myself standing by his side. I see us laughing together, showing up for each other in our dark moments, attending each other's weddings, and growing closer with each other's families. But none of that is real and I don't know why.

Why did I never come back? Why did we lose so many years?

The next morning, I put on my flannel-lined jeans, down jacket, and heavy winter boots, and walk away from our home. Since I hung up the phone with Patrick, I've been thinking of our call and little else.

My path leads me down quiet residential streets, then through the campus of St. Thomas University, a place that always reminds me of Xavier and my college years. On the other side of the campus, I follow a path into a wooded ravine. The snow crunches below my feet, and soon I arrive at the end of my journey—a cliffside overlooking the Mississippi River. Below me, the river is completely frozen. Above, the sky is gray. And, despite being in the middle of a large metropolitan area, the river bluffs are undeveloped, so I can see nothing but trees and ice.

Standing there, with nature's beauty spread before me and the powerful Mississippi frozen in place, all I can think of is Patrick—so I remove my cell phone from my pocket, take a picture, and text it to Patrick.

I write: "I walked down to the frozen Mississippi River this morning and thought of you the whole way. It was so good to hear your voice."

After sending it, I return my phone to my pocket and the dormant power of our friendship overwhelms me. All the amazing things I've seen and done since my diagnosis flash before me, and all of it—every last thing—comes with a shard of loneliness from not having shared it with Patrick, nothing except a picture of this frozen river. There is nothing to do about it but weep, so I do, and it's a long time before I stop.

Chapter 12

APRIL 14, 2004

CINCINNATI, OHIO

My cell phone rang. I was standing on campus in front of Bellarmine Chapel.

"Adam," my mom said, "I'm going to pick you up in the afternoon so we can talk."

"There is nothing to be concerned about," I assured her. "I'm fine, but if you want to talk, I'll talk."

Hours later, Farid was back by my side. I was thirsty and needed a beer. We walked into the liquor store a block from my apartment. When I put a twelve-pack of Budweiser on the counter, he took out his wallet and paid. A wave of love swept through me. I loved that man, and obviously, he loved me too.

Farid walked me back to my apartment and we parted ways. Soon after, I heard the buzzer. From my window, I could see that my mom hadn't come alone—she was with my dad, Jessica, and Kristin. I let them in. They walked up the two flights of stairs to my apartment, opened the door, stepped through, and closed the door behind them.

They told me they were there to help me, that something was wrong, and that they were going to take me to the hospital.

I told them to leave. I did not need help. Nothing was wrong. I wasn't going to the hospital. But they refused to leave.

"Get the hell out of here!" I yelled.

They ignored me.

So, I decided to ignore them. I grabbed a beer and stormed back to my bedroom, slamming the door behind me.

They tried to talk to me through the door, but I cranked up the volume on my stereo, playing Alicia Keys to drown them out. Then they tried to pry the door open, but I grabbed the knob and held them off.

They gave up, and for a while, things were calm in the apartment. They huddled in the living room. I was barricaded in my bedroom, where the music was so loud the police had to announce their arrival by shouting through my bedroom door.

Relieved that they were there, I let them in.

The two police officers and I stood in the narrow space between my single bed and my desk. Their utility belts bulged. They asked if I would turn down the music, and I did.

Methodically, I explained the situation. My family was trespassing, and I wanted them to leave.

The officers looked at the beer bottle, still full, sitting on my windowsill. They looked at each other, then they returned to the living room and informed my unwelcome guests they were trespassing.

My father told the police that, because he paid the rent, he had every right to be there (a slight fabrication since he only managed the education fund from my grandfather). The officers stood there, nonplussed. Frustrated by their inexperience and impotence, my father told them to leave.

Then my parents sent in my sister.

At that point, Jessica was the only one of them I would talk to. Up until the moment she arrived at my apartment,

Jessica thought there was nothing wrong with me. Her older brother? It was unthinkable.

Here, my memory is blank. But I do know that other than the police, Jessica was the only person who entered my bedroom. She was the only person who met me in the most isolated, shut-off place I had ever been—and somehow, she coaxed me out of there. She brought me back into the world. I can't remember how she did that, but I do remember what happened next.

Back in the living room, my parents insisted that something was wrong with me. They wouldn't listen to my explanations about why I was acting the way I was. They just wouldn't listen!

I called Farid and he agreed to come to my apartment. He had been by my side. He would tell them I was fine. When he stepped through the door, he surveyed the scene and sat down on the couch.

My family didn't know Farid and he had only known me for less than a year. But over the past few days, he had been there and hadn't judged me, at least as far as I knew. Nothing he had done gave me any indication that he was worried about me or thought I was acting out of the ordinary. For much of that morning, he had been with me as I tromped around campus, holding that blue rubber ball, which I'd taken back from Kristin.

Since he had been by my side, I thought he would take my side.

Once I explained the situation, I said, "Tell them nothing is wrong with me."

He gazed at me with compassion, and in a gentle, disarming voice, said, "Adam, you need help."

I crumpled. I was shocked.

And soon he was out the door.

———

My most vivid memory from the intervention—the one that haunts me most—was the sudden thud of my hand against my mother's face.

I hit her.

Hard.

My entire body was twisted with rage. My voice was hoarse from yelling. My words seemed to be going into a vacuum. Everyone around me was asleep. No one was on my side. Especially my parents. My muscles twitched. My laughter erupted. The air was thick with tension. No one was blinking. Everyone was crying.

Thud.

———

At first, Kristin just observed the drama unfold. But something inside of her bubbled up as the frenzy climaxed. Her compassionate strength came forth.

In the kitchen, she grabbed my head and put her forehead to mine. Our eyes met and I found solace there. She told me to breathe. She demonstrated slow, long breaths, and I mimicked her.

We stood there, in the kitchen, forehead to forehead, breathing together. My heartbeat slowed. My mind relaxed. For a moment, I was present.

———

I agreed to leave my apartment and go to the hospital, only after my parents promised that afterward, they would buy me a Stella scooter I had recently become infatuated with.

I had seen the Stellas—sleek machines modeled after the vintage Vespa scooters—at a store three blocks from my apartment. The red one called out to me. The sales clerk had told me a few days earlier that they got one hundred miles per gallon. I could feel the air brushing past my face. But first, the hospital.

We walked down the two flights of stairs and out onto the driveway, where Keady, an ex-girlfriend, stood holding a Wendy's bag. I forgot I had called her earlier and told her that I hadn't eaten for a couple days. Concerned, she showed up with my favorite fast-food option—two Wendy's spicy chicken sandwiches. My sister grabbed the bag as we got in the family van, leaving Keady standing in the driveway. Kristin stayed behind as well.

My parents headed toward Good Samaritan Hospital, where they hoped I would be admitted and given treatment, but I had other ideas. I had only promised to go *to* the hospital, not go *into* the hospital. My sister devoured a sandwich. I should have eaten one too, but my mouth was too busy filling the van with noise. I ranted and raved. Yelled and screamed. Harassed and accused. And pleaded my case.

My parents and sister were silent for the first time since appearing at my apartment. Their silence was complete. They just looked ahead with weary eyes.

When we pulled into the hospital parking lot, I opened the door and tried to bolt. The hospital was close to Farid's apartment, and I figured he would give me refuge. Certainly he had only said I needed help because of my family's presence. He knew I was fine. As quickly as I jumped out of the van, my father was out as well.

He grabbed my arm.

I tried to yank my arm away, but he wouldn't let go. I fought him, but he wouldn't let go. I yelled at him, and people turned to look, but he wouldn't let go.

With all his strength, he dragged me by the arm toward the entrance to the emergency room. Mania and my father were locked in battle in the hospital parking lot, with my life in the hands of the victor.

He wouldn't let go. And his grip was stronger than the grip of insanity.

Chapter 13

JANUARY 3, 2023

St. Paul, Minnesota

"Maybe we should talk about that," Dr. Fossum says when I describe how my father had to drag me into the hospital.

"Yeah," I say, but then say no more.

What I really need to talk about isn't that day, but another day, eight years later, when my father and I talked about the experience for the first time. So, I tell Dr. Fossum about our hiking trip to Zion Canyon.

After a day huffing up switchback trails, we sat at a table in Arkansas Al's Restaurant in the Majestic View Lodge, looking out a picture window at the vast canyon.

The setting sun danced on the warm faces of massive sandstone cliffs—cream, pink, and red—towering above the Virgin River that had eroded the cliffs at a pace only God can comprehend. Sitting there, gazing out the window, we were in the presence of the divine. My father spoke to me that night, over dinner and beers, as if God sat there with us. He opened his heart as if in prayer.

We spoke of mental illness.

He told me about a good friend, Mary, one of the first friends my parents made when they moved to Cincinnati in 1976. They moved into a four-unit apartment building on

Winding Way, just down the street from Xavier University. New to the city and knowing almost no one, they knocked on their neighbors' doors and the people they met became their first friends. Mary was one of those neighbors.

Mary was fun—lots of fun. She also had bipolar disorder.

Mary would always be fun, but over the next twenty-five years, her bipolar disorder became more severe, and her moments of fun became rarer and briefer. During that time, my father was a central figure in her support system.

Mary would sometimes come to his law office when she was going manic, talking of suing people or of conspiracies raging only in her head. My father's office manager handled Mary gracefully, making sure she got to my father so she could get help—whether that was a doctor's visit, hospitalization, or just getting her basic needs met.

As he told me this, I could see he treated her during manic episodes as he always did, as a neighbor and friend. He treated her with an eager tenderness that would heal the sickest of people if the world was a fairer place. But there were scary moments, he told me, such as when Mary wandered into the middle of four-lane Montgomery Road in the dark of night, cars whizzing by.

Mary was always around for big days throughout my childhood. She gave us a pinch to grow an inch on our birthdays, shared her gratitude at our Thanksgiving table, and forked through her Swedish rice pudding looking for the good-luck almond on Christmas Eve. I knew she was different in some ways—she moved with the noticeable slowness of the heavily drugged—but until he told me at dinner that day overlooking the cliffs, I didn't know about her bipolar disorder or the role my father played in her life.

Mary died of an overdose. Some people think she died by suicide.

My father—who was close to her, believes she always loved life, knew she was confused and often didn't understand her medication regimen—believes it was an accident. Either way, it was hard, and it was caused by her bipolar disorder.

My father was her lifeline. He felt responsible for her, treated her like family, and even wrote her obituary. He was devastated. He had no answers and lots of questions.

Less than a year later, I went manic.

My father faced the giant cliffs, but he looked back in time, to my manic episode in college. He described the day they took me to the hospital. His account was detailed, shockingly vivid, and laced with emotion.

I knew where the story was going. I had my own vivid recollections. The day of the intervention was a life-changing one for both of us and for our entire family. But, for the most part, we carried our memories in silence.

As he spoke, we were transported from Zion Canyon to the parking lot of Good Samaritan Hospital. My father's hand was gripping my arm. I was yelling at him, ordering him to release me. His jaw was clenched. His body was flexed with determination. His heart was breaking.

And then we were back at the restaurant table. My father took off his glasses and set them on the table. His face tightened as the memory of that moment overwhelmed him. Tears filled his eyes, and with a raspy voice, he said, "That was the hardest thing I have ever done."

The hardest thing he had ever done. It was the first time he told me that. The words hung in the air.

My insides twisted. I couldn't help but feel like a sense-less idiot who had lost all control and caused so much pain. I was speechless.

I knew he held no grudges. I knew our relationship had moved on. We had healed, and we had shared care-free adventures since that day. I knew that we both looked back on that day as a struggle against mental illness, not a struggle between each other.

But it was really hard to hear that the most difficult thing my father had ever done was fight me. All I wanted at that moment was to be forgiven.

As if he knew that, my dad lifted his beer and tipped it toward me. We toasted, took a sip, and he said, "Adam, I love you."

A decade later, as I tell Dr. Fossum about this conver-sation—about how dragging me into the hospital was the hardest thing my father had ever done—I am once again in tears, and she hands me a tissue.

Dr. Fossum is quiet for a moment. And then she says, "You have a tendency to take on a lot of responsibility in relationships."

I look into her eyes.

"That may have been one of the hardest things your father has ever done, but it may have also been one of his proudest moments as a parent. He got his son help."

I am silent. Disoriented—as if my personal history is getting rewritten.

Where I only saw pain and suffering stemming from my manic episode, I now see a father's pride, a shred of hope, the power of love, and the force of courage.

Since my episode, I have learned how my community pulled together to help me. Patrick drove to my parents' house one morning to tell them what he was witnessing. Kristin and my parents consulted on what to do. My parents reached out to many professionals to figure out what hospital to take me to and strategize how to do so. Farid stayed by my side to keep me safe during my mania.

Yes, my manic episode was a challenge, but many people met that challenge—eventually, even me.

<u>EMERGENCY ROOM REPORT</u>

Michelle Evanko, MD
4/14/2004

HISTORY OF PRESENT ILLNESS: The patient is a twenty-one-year-old male who was brought in by his mother and father because of irrational behavior. They believe that he has gone manic, and this is the first time that this has occurred. For the last several weeks, apparently, the patient has not been sleeping much at all. In fact, he states that he has not slept in the last three days at all. He has not been eating well either. The patient has been having irrational thoughts and behaviors. He has been spending an excessive amount of money and running up his credit card. He has given his computer away. He has talked a lot about death. His family states that he is essentially alienating most of his friends as well as his girlfriend. The patient has been very resistant to obtaining any help. His girlfriend called the parents today and they came to his apartment for the first time in a long time. When the parents arrived, apparently, he became very angry and hit both his mother and father. The patient has never had violent tendencies in the past. They feel that he is at risk of hurting other people. Apparently, he has also held down his girlfriend on the floor and hit her. At times, the patient actually has no recollection of this and states that he cannot believe that he may have forgotten this, but he believes that he could have done it. Initially, the patient was very resistant to coming into the Emergency Department to be evaluated. However, with some gentle coaxing, he did agree to talk to me. The patient does have obvious flights of ideas and very rapid speech. He cannot explain his behavior but basically states that he has been in love and that this is why he has been acting crazy. The patient denies being suicidal or homicidal. However, he admits that he really needs some sleep and cannot get it. The patient has no explanation for why he may have hit his girlfriend. He states that he hit his parents because they were trespassing in his apartment. He states he would do some family counseling. When questioned about his abnormal behavior, he does not seem to recognize that this is abnormal.

MEDICAL DECISION MAKING: This is a twenty-one-year-old male who presents in an obvious manic state. He does not appear to be acutely psychotic, and he is not truly homicidal or suicidal. However, he does have very poor impulse control and he has shown violent behavior toward others during his manic episode and does not seem to have enough impulse control to stop this. Reportedly, he has held his girlfriend down and punched her as well as his parents, which is unusual for him. He has not slept or eaten; therefore, he is not taking care of his basic needs and does not recognize the importance of getting help in order to be able to do this. I felt, given these findings, that he would qualify for a seventy-two-hour hold in order to try seeking psychiatric help. His parents also feel that he would benefit greatly from admission to the hospital. In fact, they have been in touch with the college psychologist as well as the primary physician from Xavier. A seventy-two-hour hold will be done.

Chapter 14

APRIL 14−16, 2004
CINCINNATI, OHIO

The automatic doors of the emergency room closed behind us. My parents went to the triage desk while I looked for a hidden spot to make a call. There was a low wall in the waiting room, and I sat in a chair behind it, just out of view of my parents. I knew who to call—Becca—one of my oldest friends and a friendship predating conscious memory. I had shown up for her during hard times and was certain she would show up for me.

She answered, and I got right to the point.

"Hello, Becca. I'm in the emergency room at Good Samaritan Hospital. My parents brought me here. Will you come get me out?"

A nurse approached and asked me to come with her. I hung up the phone, certain I would soon be rescued.

The nurse took me to a sterile room—two chairs, an exam table, and a countertop filled with medical supplies. My mom sat in one chair, and I sat in another, while my dad and Jessica stood across the room. The nurse asked for a urine sample.

My eyes narrowed: "Why do you want my urine? It's mine."

Next, she asked to do a blood draw.

"Now you want my blood! Ha!"

Suddenly everything crystallized. The root of all these events rocketed into my mind. There I was as a young child lying in bed, my dad beside me, and he was telling me a story as he did almost every night. The story was about a kid named Adam who went on all sorts of adventures and faced all sorts of challenges but who always succeeded, always saved the day, and always came out on top. All of what was happening in that hospital room and everything leading up to it was caused by those stories.

"Dad," I said. "Don't you see? It's because you told me those stories as a kid. Those stories about Adam."

His face betrayed him—he didn't understand.

Why did nobody understand? Why did I have to explain everything!

A large security guard came into the room and asked for my wallet and phone.

"No," I said, clasping my hands over my pockets.

He took a step toward me, "Please give me your wallet and your phone."

We stared at each other. He took another step closer and put out his hand. My urine, my blood, my phone, my wallet—they wanted it all. They wanted everything.

The security guard stood firm. No one in the room seemed at all concerned by what they were asking of me. No one was there to support me. Outnumbered, I handed over my phone and wallet.

People came and went. They asked questions, and I tried to explain. They seemed to listen, but then they would leave the room, and I wasn't released. The charade was tiring.

God, was I tired. I hadn't slept in days. When I shared this with one of the doctors, she said there was a comfortable bed upstairs. I could picture it—soft, inviting, and most importantly, away from these people and away from my family. Everyone would leave me alone, and I could lie down and sleep.

"Okay," I said, "Take me to a bed."

The elevator stopped at the tenth floor. We exited and passed through a heavy door with a small window. My dad and I sat at a table in a common area with a male nurse who began asking questions. He was wearing a cast on his arm, and my dad asked why. The nurse looked downward, his expression darkening.

Why, Dad? Why would you ask him about an injury? Why not ask him what he loves or what he finds beautiful?

I wanted my parents to leave, and after filling out some forms, they finally did.

My hospital room was simple—a bed, a cabinet, a desk, and a bathroom. The bed had a nice bounce when I pushed down on it with my palms. I kicked off my shoes, pulled back the sheets, laid down, and put my head on the pillow.

One breath and I knew something was wrong. The bed didn't feel right. It was missing something vital: the sheepskin my Aunt Kathy had given me. My body relaxed with the mere thought of its soft warm fluff creeping up along my sides. The only way I would be able to sleep was lying on that sheepskin.

I sat up in the bed. It was time to go.

I left my room and walked down the hallway to the door through which we had entered. The nurses followed me with their eyes as I passed their station. My fingers wrapped around the door handle, and I pulled. It didn't budge. I tried again. Nothing.

That's curious.

I turned and walked to the exit door at the other end of the hallway. Also locked.

There was one more door, down at the other end of the T-shaped ward. The nurses eyed me again as I passed them. When I reached the last door and pulled on the door handle, it wouldn't budge either.

Huh.

I returned to the nurses' desk and asked why the doors were locked.

"This is a secure psychiatric wing," a nurse said. "You have been involuntarily hospitalized. You are on a seventy-two-hour hold. This booklet lists your rights."

My eyes widened. My heart quickened.

WHAT THE FUCK!

At a table in the common area, I urgently flipped through the booklet. I studied it line by line, searching for a way out. Each sentence sent my mind whirling, forming arguments and building a case. One page after another, I fed the thin booklet into my seething mind.

Then I noticed something. On the wall around the corner from the nurses' station was a phone and patients were using it. My spirit soared—there was a way out!

As soon as the phone was free, I lifted it from the receiver and began dialing, calling every number I could remember and pleading with friend after friend to come and get me out of the hospital. Between calls, I sat at a table and watched the door through which I had entered, waiting for it to open and waiting for a friend.

Outside, the sun set; the streetlights flickered on; traffic died down; families sat down to dinner; and then couples crawled into bed curled together, sharing their warmth. Inside, dinner trays were wheeled into the ward; patients ate their food and shuffled off to their rooms; the fluorescent lights dimmed; and my eyes never left the door.

As night deepened, I paced the halls. All I could think about was Kristin.

She was the one person I couldn't call. The patient phone only dialed local numbers and her cell phone was long-distance. There were two nurses behind the desk, and I needed them. They were there to help, I told myself, and I needed their help.

A memory surfaced from high school. My friend Chuck and I were in the ticket line at a movie theater. On a whim, I turned to him and said, "I'm going to get us free popcorn."

He brightened and said, "Okay, let's see it."

At the ticket counter, a young woman rang up our tickets and then asked if we would like anything from concessions.

"Yes," I said, "We'd like free popcorn."

She smiled. "Well, I can't do that."

I smiled and tilted my head to the side.

"Well, what if I did a freestyle rap right now, just for you, could we get free popcorn then?"

It was the late nineties, the golden age of hip-hop—Snoop, Outkast, Dr. Dre, The Notorious B.I.G.—a personal freestyle rap was irresistible to any high schooler in America.

"Okay." She chuckled.

A couple of minutes later, Chuck and I were watching a terrible Batman movie, munching away on free popcorn.

As I approached the nurses' desk, I summoned the irresistible charm that could get me whatever I wanted.

My voice filled with genuine need, I asked, "Would you please let me use your cell phone?"

The closest nurse looked up.

"I need to call my girlfriend and her cell phone has a different area code."

The nurse smiled, making my heart leap, but then said, "I'm sorry, but I can't do that."

I smiled in return and cranked up the charm. I told her our love story, how I was concerned about Kristin, how it would just take a moment, and how our relationship depended on it.

No.

My charm evaporated, and I began to beg.

No.

I negotiated.

No.

I blamed.

No.

I spat.

No.

And then the sun came up.

I returned to the patient phone and continued to canvass my friends.

Not long after, an orderly approached. My friends and family called the hospital, concerned by the calls I was making. My phone privileges were revoked. No more calls.

"What! Are you fucking kidding?"

He wasn't.

My only line of communication with the outside world had been cut. My world had shrunk to the tenth floor of Good Samaritan Hospital.

No one listened to me.

Not the nurses. Not the doctors. My life was in their hands, and they refused to listen, but I wasn't going silently.

They wouldn't take away my voice. They took away my freedom but never my voice.

Pacing the halls of the ward, I remembered *Amistad*, and I remembered Joseph Cinque.

Shortly before my manic episode, I watched *Amistad*, Steven Spielberg's film about Joseph Cinque and a group of West Africans who were kidnapped and sold into slavery in 1836. They revolted onboard their slave ship, killing their captors and winding up in an American courtroom, facing a jury charged with deciding whether they were property or free men.

My plight paled in comparison to theirs, but a scene in the movie hit me as I paced the halls. My eyes narrowed as I headed toward the nurses' station.

In the film, Cinque interrupts the court proceedings, whispering, "Give us, us free," publicly speaking English for the first time.

A few people turn their heads toward him.

"Give us, us free," he says louder as he stands.

The district attorney appeals to the judge. "Please instruct the defendant that he cannot disrupt these proceedings with such outburs—."

"Give us, us free!" Cinque yells, extending his chained arms in front of him toward the judge.

The judge bangs his gavel, but the whole courtroom is now under Cinque's spell. The passion and longing and injustice in Cinque's simple expression overwhelm everyone watching.

Cinque crescendos, "GIVE US, US FREE!"

I stood in front of the nurses' station, wearing light blue hospital pajamas and glaring at the staff behind the desk.

They ignored me. They ignored my fury. I had been captured against my will, brought to this hospital, and locked behind closed doors. I wasn't a slave, stripped of my homeland and all my human rights, but I was a prisoner. These people were my jailers.

I whispered, "Let me free."

Nothing.

I said it louder, "Let me free!"

They just typed on their keyboards and flipped through their files.

"Let Me Free!" I shouted.

A couple of heads turned my way.

"LET ME FREE!" I thundered.

Everyone at the nurses' station stopped what they were doing and looked at me. I fixed them with a scowl and waited to be led to the door.

"You need to calm down," said a nurse. They returned to their work, and I went back to pacing the halls.

The day passed. Then another night, moving between my room, the halls, and the common area. Thinking. Planning. Fuming.

The next morning, Dr. Nunlist-Young arrived during breakfast as I walked the halls with an individual-sized box of Cheerios in my hands. I plucked Cheerio after Cheerio out of the box and popped it into my mouth. Despite having eaten nearly nothing for six days, I was unbothered by my starved stomach. The series of injustices perpetrated against me crowded out all other concerns.

Dr. Nunlist-Young was my family doctor and treated me throughout my life.

Seeing him confused me. *What was he doing there?*

Immediately, I was on him, questioning his presence. While I interrogated him, he scribbled on a clipboard held close to his chest.

Enough with this bullshit, this secrecy.

I asked him to show me his clipboard. He just looked at me.

I demanded to see his clipboard. He stammered out a few words. Large male orderlies wandered over and began hovering nearby. Dr. Nunlist-Young pulled his clipboard closer to his chest. Like everyone in the world, it seemed he couldn't care less about what I wanted or about my liberty, my rights, my thoughts, and me.

I shot out my right arm, wrapped my fingers around the top of his clipboard, and began yanking it. Dr. Nunlist-Young's eyes widened. He clamped down on the clipboard and pulled it closer to his chest. For a brief moment, we engaged in a tug-of-war, but then the orderlies grabbed me by the arms. There were a lot of them, more than I could handle.

They lifted me off my feet and carried me around the corner as I screamed, kicked, and struggled. They carried me into a small room and shut the door behind us. There was a bed in the middle of the room, low to the ground, padded with a vinyl cover but no sheets. At its corners were heavy straps.

The orderlies set me down on my feet next to the bed, then fanned out around the room. They were on edge, tense, and serious. I, on the other hand, thought this entire situation was absurd. I was already being held against my will; now they were going to strap me down? *Ludicrous, simply ludicrous.*

The orderly across the bed said, "If you don't calm down and stop lashing out at people, we're going to put you in restraints." He paused. "Can you calm down and behave peacefully?"

I smiled and looked at this frightened man. He was large, muscular, sharp-eyed, and wearing white hospital garb.

Does he think that will scare me?

He didn't know me. He didn't understand. He was just another cog in the wheel of the forces against me.

I looked at his companions in the room, all similarly large and tense, and realized I stood no chance. I was totally at their mercy. I couldn't out-muscle these guys. But I still had my box of Cheerios.

A thought flew into my head, and it was beautiful, unavoidable, and compelling.

Fuck these guys. They won't break me.

I reached into my box, extracted a single Cheerio, and cradled it between my fingers. I looked through the hole at the bed, noticed the tiny air pockets speckling the cereal, then pulled my arm back and threw the Cheerio at the orderly's face.

I caught him off guard. He hadn't expected a Cheerio attack. I reached back into the box and threw another, with roaring laughter erupting from somewhere deep within me.

After another Cheerio hit, the orderly took a deep breath and lowered his chin. He made eye contact with his companions, and they closed in on me. From all sides, they seized me and slammed me down on the bed.

Cheerios went flying everywhere. I squirmed and kicked, yanking my limbs away from their grasp, flexing my muscles with all my might. But one by one, the restraints cinched down around my ankles and wrists. Those fuckers tied me down.

This didn't stop my struggle. I fought the restraints, pulling on them with all my strength. I yelled out, screaming till I went hoarse.

Never had I channeled such fury. Never had my body flexed with such might. As urgent thoughts raced through my mind, I shouted them into the room—I pledged to convert religions, demanded they stop giving my mother medicine, and pleaded for an end to my captivity.

Nurses and doctors came in to speak with me, to convince me to take medicine.

I agreed, took the pills in my mouth, and then spit them into the air only to have them land on my forehead. But after a couple hours, they wore me down and I swallowed.

As the drugs kicked in, my mind began to slow, my struggle ceased, and I surrendered to utter exhaustion.

I had been awake for 144 hours straight—six full days. Restrained and drugged, I slept for the next twenty-four hours.

Chapter 15

MARCH 5, 2019

CINCINNATI, OHIO

It was a precious evening. As the parents of young children, Geoff and I did our best to meet up in the evenings, have a beer, and talk, but our children's bedtimes and our exhaustion afterward made such evenings rare. This was back in 2019, when our children were quite young, and bedtime was an elaborate production.

We were at Sorrento's, a storied Italian restaurant and sports bar in Cincinnati that I had been going to since my childhood. There were just a few other people in the bar. We had a lot to talk about. We always have a lot to talk about, because we are the best of friends, and no subject is off limits.

He told me about his work as a township administrator, all the crazy citizens hassling him, and the crazier politicians—his bosses—with their random obsessions. He was blowing off steam to one of the few people who could fully understand. I had quit my job as an attorney a few months prior, but I used to sue government officials—people exactly like him—so I got it.

"What are you doing these days?" he asked.

I told him I was in limbo. I was no longer a lawyer and unsure of what would come next. In the evenings, I cooked for the family and played with Phoenix, who was almost three. During the days, I had picked up my memoir and was working on it again, my third go.

I paused and sipped my beer. "I've been thinking a lot about bipolar disorder."

He grew quiet. I could tell he had disappeared into a memory, and I was pretty sure which one.

Geoff was the first person to visit me in the hospital after I was released from the restraints. He hadn't seen me for weeks leading up to that moment. He attended the University of Cincinnati, a few miles from Xavier, so we didn't regularly see each other. He hadn't seen me go manic, as my college friends had, but he heard I was in the hospital, so he came to visit.

The bar around us seemed to recede. Geoff's face grew sober, ashen. He shook his head from side to side and tapped his pint absentmindedly, staring off into some void as he traveled back to that day he visited the tenth floor of Good Samaritan Hospital, a day we had never fully discussed.

He told me how he stood outside the locked door of the psychiatric ward, looking through the window into a strange world he had never seen before. Then he entered, sat with me at a table, and we talked.

I was poring over the pamphlet, explaining my rights, plotting my court strategy, and trying to understand how the hell I would get out of the hospital. I was taking psychiatric drugs for the first time in my life, and, despite twenty-four hours of sleep, I was still very manic.

He described the other patients—disheveled, drugged, and delusional. Then he described me—rigid face, serious demeanor, drugged cadence, and so much anger.

He paused and looked at the wall behind me, as if I wasn't there…as if there was a window with a vivid view of the past.

"That wasn't you, Adam. That wasn't you."

Geoff and I have been friends since seventh grade. He was there when I came of age—from when I couldn't grow a mustache up through the day I shaved "2000" into my beard for our high school graduation. When I was climbing out of my deep depression, Geoff was one of the first friends I reconnected with. Since he hadn't seen me go manic, his presence triggered joy, not terror, and so our friendship grew while my college friendships faded. We have grown incredibly close since. He can finish all my favorite stories and is featured in most. He knows me as few do—very few.

We sat in silence for a while. Then he turned and looked me directly in the eyes. "That wasn't you."

Since that night at Sorrento's, I've tried to believe Geoff. God, how I wish the person in the hospital wasn't me.

For many years I have tried and tried and tried to separate myself from that manic me who was so out of control they strapped him down like a wild beast. Every part of me wants distance from the visceral feeling of those straps digging into my wrists as I tried to tear my arms free.

For eighteen years, the trauma of my hospitalization has lingered. What was done to me, and what I did to others. The distance between myself and my community. The deep well of rage and fury that I floundered in for nearly two weeks. It was unlike any other experience in my life.

It was so strange that I sequestered it in a cache of memories belonging to someone else—someone I no longer am, someone who only existed for a blink. I keep my hospitalization as far from my self-image as possible.

But neither neglect nor conscious denial work. I'm forty years old now, and the memories persist. It's time to stop fighting it and face the truth. It's time to reconcile and be whole.

Geoff was wrong.

It was me.

Chapter 16

APRIL 17–27, 2004
CINCINNATI, OHIO

After twenty-four hours and fifteen minutes, they unstrapped my wrists and ankles, and two hours later, they let me out of the seclusion room. It was April 17, a Sunday, and my seventy-two-hour hold was scheduled to end the next day.

In Ohio, a patient could be admitted involuntarily to a psychiatric ward for seventy-two hours if a doctor deemed them a danger to themselves or others. But any involuntary hospitalization beyond that needed to be ordered by a judge—the patient had to be civilly committed. Because I was admitted on a Wednesday, and the courts were closed over the weekend, my involuntary hospitalization was actually a hold of one hundred and twenty hours.

As it was ending, my dad and the hospital staff wanted me to sign a paper to become a voluntary patient and avoid the court hearing. But I didn't give a shit what they wanted. Instead, I was building my case.

By Monday morning, I had studied the patient handbook, my defense for the hearing was taking shape, and I was gearing up for a fight. But at breakfast, something changed.

A young man entered the hospital ward and sat at one of the tables in the common area with his parents and a nurse—just as I had when I arrived. He looked around the common area with nervous eyes, which came to rest on me. We stared at each other for a moment, and then I scanned the room. The other patients were looking at me too, as if they expected something from me, something only I could do.

I took a deep breath. I got it. I suddenly realized I was needed there.

This young man needed me. He needed my guidance. He needed my help. This was why I had been tested and tortured. This was why I had been studying and learning my rights—our rights! Since I had work to do on the ward, I signed the papers and became a voluntary patient.

Afterward, back in my room, I emptied out the suitcase my parents had brought me—one of those old hard-walled suitcases like an oversized briefcase. I loaded it with the patient handbook, some paper, and crayons. Satisfied, I closed the clasps and walked out of my room.

The new patient was now alone at the table, and I strode over to him. The sound of my suitcase smacking down on his table echoed through the halls. I sat across from him and got right to business. "It looks like you need a lawyer." I opened the suitcase and removed the patient handbook.

He looked startled, but he stayed seated as I explained his rights. When I finished, he nodded, got up, and went to his room. After that, he rarely came out, and when he did, he never approached me.

———

During the remainder of my hospitalization, escape was always on my mind. I couldn't physically leave, but I could resist the powers aligned against me. I shunned the professionals and their irrelevant talk of mental illness and turned to my fellow patients for help. I most often found that help in the smoking room.

Good Samaritan Hospital had hundreds of rooms, but there was one that was like no other—the tenth-floor in-patient psychiatric smoking room.

Furnished only with three chairs and a giant ash-tray, time in the smoking room was precious and in high demand. It was the only room that was exclusively used by the patients. The nurses and doctors could watch us through a small video camera in the upper corner of the room, but unless there was some emergency, they never disturbed us. The smoking room was a refuge.

For me, it was a much-needed escape from the forces conspiring against me. In the smoking room, I could be myself—my unfiltered self—and no one judged. There were no clipboards in the smoking room. Questions weren't loaded. In the smoking room, I could relax and breathe fresh air.

The door had a small window and a sign posted on the outside listing the rules. There were two institutional rules: three patients at a time and one cigarette per visit.

But there were other rules—temporary rules, unwritten rules—that depended on the ruler. The smoking room was the patients' kingdom, and we had our kings and queens. Some were benevolent; others were fiercely angry and intolerant. And the politics were impossible to master, for each time a patient entered or left the room, the balance of power shifted.

The grizzled old man sitting across from me was a dictator. No one stood up to him. No one challenged his tyrannical power. Except me.

Tension filled the smoking room. The old man snarled at me. "I've been in and out of places like this since before you were born." His eyes narrowed. "I was in Vietnam. I killed people! And I'll kill you too if you don't stop telling me you love me!"

This was unacceptable. The man's anger polluted the room, and it could only be cleansed with love.

The woman seated between us leaned toward me and whispered, "Just be quiet."

No, I couldn't be quiet. His anger was too much. If I didn't stand up to him, it would persist and continue to spoil that sacred space.

My heart opened as I smiled and said, "I love you."

He stared at me with pure rage in his eyes as his cigarette burned down toward his fingers. But he stayed in his seat, as we all did when we were in the smoking room.

Hours later, he was wheeled from the psychiatric wing on a stretcher wearing an oxygen mask—his eyes followed me as he rolled down the hall and I knew I was the cause.

Despite occasional moments of conflict and sometimes chaos, the smoking room was the most therapeutic room in the wing.

Within its sanctuary, other patients gave me passages of the Bible to read, CDs to listen to, and brands of cigarettes to try. I followed those prescriptions with all my heart and soul, and they helped.

One day, I noticed a patient in the smoking room who seemed at peace. I watched her throughout the day and observed she constantly wore headphones attached to a CD player. When I asked what she was listening to, she wrote down the name of the CD: Carlos Nakai, *Canyon Trilogy, Volume 5.*

On my parents' next visit, I told them to buy me that CD and bring me a CD player. When they did, I listened for hours and for days. The Native American flute music possessed me. It was delicate, fragile, and filled with longing. It calmed my heartbeat, occupied my mind, and took me far away from the hospital, to canyons, mountains, and rivers.

The world around me—the nurses, the other patients, the linoleum floor, the medication regimens, and the mealtimes—disappeared. It was just me and the music.

A few days after being admitted, I discovered the refrigerator in the common area was always filled with individual cartons of milk. I found packets of graham crackers in a drawer next to it.

I began eating graham crackers and milk daily, sometimes two or three times a day. I would break up the graham crackers into a Styrofoam cup, pour milk over them, patiently wait until they had soaked up the milk, then eat the smooth delicious mush that was a Gerhardstein family delicacy, dating back generations. It was better medicine than the pills they gave me.

A week into my hospitalization, at lunch, I made another discovery—a patient at a table next to mine had two cheeseburgers.

"How did you get two cheeseburgers?"

"Haven't you noticed that slip of paper that comes on your food tray?"

"No."

"Wow. How long have you been here? Anyways, you can fill it out and they will bring you whatever you want tomorrow." He smiled and patted his belly. "You can even

write an X with a number two if you want two cheeseburgers or something."

He blew my mind. The secrets of the psych ward seemed
never-ending.

In the second week of my hospitalization, I began playing
their game. I participated in therapy groups, talked to the
psychologist, and agreed to participate in an outpatient
program once released.

The hospital granted me a few passes out of the facility for a couple hours chaperoned by my parents. While
out of the hospital on one of the earlier passes, I became
confrontational with my parents, but then, on one pass, I
controlled myself and stayed calm.

A day or two later, they wrote me a series of prescriptions, scheduled appointments with a psychiatrist and a talk
therapist, and let me go. After thirteen days in the hospital,
I was finally free.

In the hours before my release, I stood at the windows
of the common room, looking out, wondering what I was
going to do out there and how I was going to make sense
of all that had happened. My gaze settled on a convenience
store across the street. I thought of the smoking room—how
it was the one place where I felt real therapy happened.

*Maybe I could get a job at that convenience store, selling
cigarettes—dispensing medicine.*

The day after I was released, I turned in an application.

The convenience store never called.

Chapter 17

JANUARY 10, 2023
St. Paul, Minnesota

"Have I ever told you how I got naked in the hospital?" I ask Meredith.

We are on our couch, lounging at opposite ends, facing each other.

"No," she says with a slight smile.

"There are two ways of seeing what happened to me in the hospital," I tell her. "On the surface, the stories can be sort of amusing, but there's a deeper level that is more difficult to explain."

Her smile fades.

"Let me tell you what happened first. I was in my hospital room and decided to take off all my clothes. So, I got naked and walked out of my room to the nurses' station. Then I just stood there naked, staring at them."

My tone is nonchalant and Meredith's uncertain smile returns, but then my voice drops.

"But…" I pause. "What was really happening was that I was so angry. I was furious. I felt completely powerless. They had locked me up and I couldn't leave. Then I had the thought that they could take my freedom, but they couldn't make me wear clothes. So, I didn't get naked on a whim. It was an act of resistance."

For a moment, I feel that old fury. The power of compulsion. There I am, walking out of my hospital room with scorn and my head held high.

"From the outside, it looked crazy—just a naked guy walking down the hall. But in my mind, it was an act of desperation. I was very serious."

"What did the nurses do?" Meredith asks.

"They just ran out from behind the desk and led me back to my room and told me I couldn't walk around naked."

Meredith watches me, but I've drifted away from her into my memories. It's been a long time since I remembered my hospitalization in this way.

I've tried to erase the anger I felt in the hospital by telling myself that my hospitalization was necessary, that I needed help but didn't realize it, that I was sick, and that's why I acted as I did. I've tried to bury the way I felt being hospitalized.

But as I return to that moment when I walked out of my hospital room naked, I realize the feelings are still alive.

———

"There is a word coming to mind," Dr. Fossum says as I recount my conversation with Meredith. She adjusts her position in her chair.

"Power."

She lets the word fill the room.

"Do you know what I mean?"

I do. I know it deep within me. I know it underneath all those layers of embarrassment and fear. It comes to me with force, without shame, and with pure conviction.

"I had a lot of fucking fight in me."

"Yes," she says. "You had a lot of fucking fight in you."

We sit with that for a moment.

"And," she says, "that is something you can be proud of."

I fall back onto the couch and absorb her words. They penetrate layers of shame so thick they are calloused.

For the last eighteen years, my hospitalization has haunted me. A fright so profound that it has stunned me into near silence. Those extraordinary experiences I keep locked away from the world. But they're always there, motivating my management of bipolar disorder because I don't want to go back. Ever.

My experience in the hospital was bad enough, but, not long after my release, I made it worse by blaming myself for my hospitalization. It was me. It was my fault. I was an idiot, and I lost control. I was sick and didn't know it but somehow should have.

My hospitalization was a terrible thing to endure. I was locked up and lashed down merely because I was sick. This wasn't my fault, or my parents' fault, or even the staff at the hospital's fault. It's just the way our culture has decided to deal with humans experiencing a rare state of mind.

Is there a better way? Probably.

But when I was subjected to this form of treatment, I didn't buckle. I fought back. And for the first time, I realize there is no shame in that.

Chapter 18

APRIL 27–MAY 20, 2004
CINCINNATI, OHIO

When I was released from the hospital, I needed space. My space. It was time to move out of the apartment I shared with Patrick. He wasn't pushing me out, but I was uncomfortable sleeping in the room where the police had confronted me. The whole apartment was filled with furious memories.

Patrick was figuring out how to be a father to the child he had just learned about, and, while I was in the hospital, Patrick's father had died in Kenya. Patrick organized a memorial service at Xavier's chapel that I attended two days after leaving the hospital.

Patrick needed a friend. I needed a friend. But, at that moment, neither of us was well-equipped to be that friend. I know I wasn't.

Within a few days, I found an apartment a fifteen-minute walk down the hill from Good Samaritan Hospital—an easy commute to outpatient therapy. My uncle and cousin came down from Dayton, Ohio, in their minivan and helped me move into a third-floor, one-bedroom unit in the Clifton Colony Apartments. I signed a one-year lease. The rent was cheap, and it would be paid out of my college account until I finished school and got a job.

My outpatient therapy wasn't scheduled to begin until May 12, seventeen days after my release from the hospital. As I prepared to enter the program, I was unconvinced I was bipolar, and it nagged at me that so many others were certain of it. While I could live with the doctors' mistaken diagnosis, I needed my loved ones to see me as they always had, as I was, a mentally sound person whose behavior was grounded in reality.

I developed a plan. I would sit down with Kristin, Patrick, my parents, and Jessica and listen to them. I would invite them to tell me what their recent experience with me had been like. Then, after they had gotten it all out, I would explain everything, show them that I wasn't crazy, and that everything I had done made sense.

I began with Patrick, then Kristin, and then my parents. None of them listened to me. And hearing their perspectives took a toll on me. Jessica was my last hope.

We sat down on the front porch of our childhood home. My plan was to patiently listen to her without interruption. I knew we had very different perspectives on the last month of my life. But she was my sister; she knew me. If I could just get her to listen, then I would have at least one person on my side. But first, I knew I had to listen.

As Jessica spoke, I watched her eyes. They glanced down at the concrete floor of the porch and then out toward the street. Occasionally, she looked directly at me, into my desperation.

She told me what it was like watching our dad call the police on her brother. And then what it was like when our parents sent her into my locked bedroom where I had barricaded myself during the intervention, after the police had come and gone. She explained how she was the only person I would listen to and how my parents relied on her to coax me out.

She told me how terrifying it was when I hit our mom.

She told me she got permission from her teachers to bring her cell phone to class. She told them her brother was in a psychiatric hospital and he wouldn't talk to her parents. He would only talk to her.

She told me about the strange note I gave her when I was in the hospital, which read: "Make new stories but discard the old, for one is silver and the others gold…bling bling. I want gold trim on my scooter. And I want it to be purple (or orange)—the rest is fire. What do you think?"

She told me how we were playing "Sorry!" with our dad in the hospital, and I broke down and cried when my dad "Sorried" me.

She told me how her friends were very supportive at first but soon couldn't see that she was still hurting.

Suddenly, she went quiet. There was something else she wanted to tell me before I got my chance to explain.

I picked at the wicker chair with my fingernails, peeling off the white paint. Baby birds chirped out for lunch from their nests in the honeysuckle bushes along the driveway. My mother's daffodils trumpeted toward the sun.

Jessica took a deep breath.

"This was supposed to be my time," she murmured.

She looked up at me with the saddest eyes. Eyes that had seen fate destroy her expectations. Her very reasonable expectations.

She would soon graduate from Walnut Hills High School, one of the most challenging academic experiences in Ohio, and every one of her report cards had been flawless. All As. A 4.0 GPA. An amazing accomplishment. And now, all she wanted was to have that accomplishment recognized. She wanted to finish high school with a bang, with our family's focus on her. She deserved it.

But during the last month, as she took her final exams, planned her graduation party, and picked up her cap and gown, our family's attention was elsewhere. She was an afterthought. As she looked forward to her graduation celebrations, she knew that my manic episode and our family's pain would be a dark cloud, casting a shadow on what she had hoped to be a season of joy. The proper time to pause and celebrate her hard work turned out to be all about Adam.

My sister's eyes are easy to read, for me, perhaps, better than anyone.

I have seen them long for friendship, shed tears of disappointment, flash with anger, laugh with joy, and widen in curiosity. They've told me about her first boyfriends, at first seeking advice, then sharing bliss and heartache. They've sought pep talks before ice-skating competitions and solace after falling in front of the judges. Over eighteen years, her eyes had told me the story of her childhood, but that changed on the porch that day.

Jessica had seen things her friends never had. Things most people never see. She had confronted mania in its purest form. Unchecked. Untreated. Unexpected. Her eyes were no longer those of a child.

I had never seen those eyes before. They were scared, not of the moment, but of the future. They searched me for some sign that I would come back to her.

Suddenly, I saw the broken moment. I saw myself celebrating her—toasting her in the cleverest way at the finest restaurant in Cincinnati, giving her a hand-drawn book telling the story of her glory. She was laughing. Joyous. Being idolized by her older brother.

In her eyes, I saw the person I hadn't been, the person she expected me to be, the person I thought I was. Her eyes searched me for some sign I was still that person, that there was some hope I would snap out of it and raise a glass to my amazing sister.

I looked into her eyes and saw the truth.

Truth comes in many forms, but when it appears–when it truly appears–there is no arguing with it.

Jessica had given up trying to convince me of anything. But there was an unavoidable truth in her confession. Suddenly, I could see her capstone moment cracking and her hopes crumbling. She was making her peace with it, but it was painful, and I could not argue with her pain. I could only feel it as only a brother can.

I heard a whisper within—a questioning that would only grow louder in the weeks ahead.

Am I wrong about all of this?

Is something wrong with me?

———

A few days later, I walked up the hill to my first day in the outpatient therapy program. It was on the tenth floor of Good Samaritan Hospital, right across the hall from the locked door leading into the psychiatric ward where I had been hospitalized.

Cognitive behavioral therapy, art therapy, talk therapy— none of it resonated. There was no denying my life had changed—that something powerful had happened. My family and friends encouraged me to accept I was sick. The outpatient program was premised on the notion that I had a mental illness or, at least, that I had ways of thinking that I should change and issues I needed to address. This premise was problematic.

My mind had fueled my entire life—a beautiful life—and my thinking over the last month felt no different than all the months before. It felt equally real. Neither psychotic nor delusional. I had reasons for all my actions, and my thoughts had been profound. But no one understood, and no one would listen.

Instead, they wanted me to listen and accept that my mind was broken. Whenever that possibility crept into my thinking, I felt a flash of absolute devastation. So, I pushed it away.

The cognitive behavioral group therapist had an annoying habit of bending forward in his chair, pulling up his slacks, and then stretching his knee-length socks up his legs. When he would leave the room, I impersonated him—much to the delight of my fellow patients. In art therapy, when I made a mask for one of our assignments, the therapist asked, "Do you feel like you are wearing a mask?" The anger I felt during my hospitalization bubbled up as my defenses snapped into place. *Who is this therapist? She doesn't know me!*

After one week, I had had enough. The program staff reminded me I had just gotten out of the hospital and this program would help me from going back, so I should stay. But I couldn't spend one more day at Good Samaritan Hospital. I withdrew from the program on my twenty-second birthday.

That night I drove to my parents' house in my Dodge Neon but expected to drive home on the sleek red scooter with chrome trim they had promised me during the intervention at my apartment.

When I parked in front of their house, I looked down the driveway to see if the scooter was there—nothing, but maybe it was in the garage.

For most of my birthdays throughout my youth, my family ate dinner at Sorrento's, came home, and sat at the kitchen table to eat lemon poppyseed cake as I opened my presents.

On my twenty-second birthday, though, when it came time for gifts, we didn't sit around the table eating cake. No, it was just my parents and me, standing in my mother's office, a small room off the kitchen. Despite it being a cramped space for three people, there was a great distance between us. When my father gave me my birthday card, it felt like I had to walk a mile to take it from his hand.

There were two possibilities. Either that card said there was a scooter in the garage waiting for me, or it didn't. Either the promise they had made was real, or it was a lie. Either they had taken me seriously, or they hadn't.

The promise of that scooter helped me endure my hospitalization. When I was locked up in the psychiatric ward, the image of myself zipping through the city, with the wild breeze all around me, was the ultimate fantasy of freedom.

A scooter wasn't hidden in the garage. My birthday gift was that my parents would credit me $500 on my credit card debt.

I didn't stay long.

To celebrate my birthday, I took myself to the movies. I walked up the hill from my new apartment to the Esquire

Theater, Cincinnati's destination for independent films and documentaries.

I bought one ticket, a tub of popcorn, and a Coke. There were only a few other people in the theater watching the last movie on a Thursday night. Going to the movies alone was exciting, a first for me. It felt like a unique way to celebrate a birthday.

I watched *Super Size Me*, a documentary about the fast-food industry and a man who ate nothing but McDonald's for thirty days straight, a diet that wrecked his health and also planted a seed in the back of my mind.

After the movie ended, I walked along Ludlow Avenue, peering into the shop windows until I came to Uno's Chicago Pizzeria a few doors down. Its restaurant was tucked into the basement, but its bar was at ground level, with large windows overlooking the street. *Yes*, I thought, *time for a celebratory birthday drink*. Another first—going to a bar alone.

Dr. Gupta, the psychiatrist I had reluctantly seen since getting out of the hospital, advised me not to drink alcohol—it's a depressant and could destabilize my mood. But I was twenty-two and had been closing down the bars with Patrick since I was nineteen. Giving up alcohol felt like I would be giving up on having fun. That wasn't going to happen.

"I'll have a whiskey and ginger."

The bartender eyed me.

"Can I see an ID?"

I took my wallet out of my rear pocket and slid out my driver's license. As the bartender inspected my ID, I smiled and announced, "It's my birthday."

He looked up with the exuberant smile that restaurant employees perfect for that moment as if hearing that news is the highlight of their shift. But as he opened his mouth to say, "Happy Birthday," his eyes darted to either side of me. I deflated.

I knew what he was looking at—the empty space around me—and I knew how that looked.

When he said, "Happy Birthday," he said something different with his eyes.

Earlier that day, I had walked out of Good Samaritan Hospital defiant and determined. But this bartender caught me with my defenses down. It was late and I was tired. The fight had left me.

I didn't respond to the bartender's judgment by building up my rationale, crafting my narrative, or preparing to explain why I was alone and proud of it. Instead, I quietly paid for my drink and sat at a circular high-top table by the window.

Alone on my birthday, I felt my hope that I was still normal slipping away. My resistance to my diagnosis was collapsing.

Dr. Gupta had recently said, "You had a textbook manic episode."

I tried not to hear him, but then he explained what the textbook said.

The *Diagnostic and Statistical Manual of Mental Disorders*, which he called the DSM, said that a manic episode is defined as "a distinct period of abnormally and persistently elevated, expansive, or irritable mood, lasting at least one week."

But what I had been through wasn't so abnormal; everything had seemed to make sense.

Then Dr. Gupta got down to specifics. During that period of mood disturbance, he told me that at least three of seven symptoms must have persisted:

1. "Inflated self-esteem is typically present, ranging from uncritical self-confidence to marked grandiosity, and may reach delusional proportions."
   Well, I had been convinced my thoughts killed my grandfather.

2. "Almost invariably, there is a decreased need for sleep."
   How many nights had I gone without sleeping? Was it five or six?

3. "Speech is typically pressured, loud, rapid, and difficult to interrupt. Individuals may talk nonstop, sometimes for hours on end, and without regard for others' wishes to communicate."
   The faces of the staff of the Newswire *were quite shocked as I confronted the editor. I suppose I was rather loud and felt an urgency that was a bit much.*

4. "The individual's thoughts may race, often at a rate faster than can be articulated."
   The letter I wrote to Kristin about our grandparents was all over the place, and she seemed lost when I tried to explain it to her.

5. "Distractibility is evidenced by an inability to screen out irrelevant external stimuli. There may be a reduced ability to differentiate between thoughts that are germane to the topic and thoughts that are only slightly relevant or clearly irrelevant."
   There was that shuttle ride, when I was so tired and wanted to sleep but was suddenly compelled to save the driver's job. And that letter to Father Graham... what was the point of all those things about my college experience?

6. "Increase in goal-directed activity often involves excessive planning of, and excessive participation in, multiple activities."
The months before I stopped sleeping were rather busy. My work with Ugali, leading a spiritual retreat, the series of articles for the Newswire, *and writing a manifesto of a term paper. I had taken on quite a bit.*

7. "Expansiveness, unwarranted optimism, grandiosity, and poor judgment often lead to an imprudent involvement in pleasurable activities such as buying sprees, reckless driving, foolish business investments, and sexual behavior unusual for the person, even though these activities are likely to have painful consequences."
My credit card bill. Driving drunk. My road trip flings with two women even though Kristin and I were in the early stages of a long-desired romance. I certainly hadn't been making the best choices.

The DSM continued beyond those symptoms: "The disturbance must be sufficiently severe to cause marked impairment in social or occupational functioning or to require hospitalization, or it is characterized by the presence of psychotic features."

And there I was—at a bar alone on my birthday, behind in my college courses, not far removed from a thirteen-day hospitalization, during which my psychiatrist was saying I was psychotic.

In the quiet, nearly empty bar, Dr. Gupta's voice wasn't the only one I heard. The stories of my loved ones echoed within me. I couldn't unhear the conversations I had initiated. And their experiences were so different than my own. Not just what they saw me do, but how my behavior made them feel and how they still felt. The distance between us was still growing.

I had pushed away everyone who loved me as I clung to the hope that I wasn't bipolar, while actively resisting really knowing what it meant. All I wanted to do was hide from my diagnosis, from everyone who had seen me manic, and from my overwhelming fear that I was at the beginning of a long, rocky road into a dismal future.

I looked out the window at Ludlow Avenue. The street was calm. No pedestrians walked the sidewalk. Only a few cars drove by. The shops were closed, and the lights were off.

It was just me and my drink.

Chapter 19

JANUARY 17, 2023
St. Paul, Minnesota

It's midway through our session when my memories of those conversations after my hospitalization surface. I stop talking and sit in silence for a moment.

"Shortly after I got out of the hospital," I say to Dr. Fossum, "I decided to have conversations with my parents, my sister, Patrick, and Kristin. My plan was to listen to them and their experience of my manic episode, so that then they would hopefully listen to me, and I could explain that everything made sense."

Dr. Fossum lets out a sympathetic sigh.

"Listening to their stories was really hard." My body clenches up. "Seeing myself through their eyes was painful."

I'm not crying, but I'm close. From the way Dr. Fossum looks at me, I see I don't need to go any further. She understands. I stop speaking and sit with my memories.

"Do you think you were ready to have those conversations?" she asks.

Damn, what a question, and I am not ready to answer it. I mumble a few things, filling the silence while the question burrows into my story.

That afternoon, as I move through the day, my thoughts never leave the memory of those conversations. They were my idea. I brought them on myself. They happened, so what does it matter if I was ready?

When I wake the next day, the question still lingers. I have breakfast, sit down to write, edit a few chapters, and then go for a walk. It's a gray winter day, without a glimmer of sunshine and nothing to pull my attention away from my thoughts.

Looking down at the icy sidewalk, I suddenly understand why it's such a difficult question to answer: it isn't really a question. Dr. Fossum was suggesting something I may have never had the humility to admit—I wasn't ready to have those conversations.

A layer of my foundation crumbles.

The many years of telling myself how important those conversations were and how they helped me along the path of acceptance of my diagnosis now seem like deceit. At a visceral level, I know but have never had the strength to admit that this narrative is partial—true, but partial.

The helpfulness of those conversations obscures how much I hated them and how I always will. They were painful. My loved ones had vastly different experiences during my mania than I did. Through their eyes, I saw that difference. Through their mouths, I heard my words. Through their tears, I felt the trauma my behavior caused.

As defiant as I was, their experiences got to me—and damn, I was just days out of the hospital.

A week after Dr. Fossum asked that question, I finally get it: it is time to let go.

Now, eighteen years since those conversations, it's time to drop the load of my loved ones' pain.

Just as I must live with bipolar disorder, they must love someone who has bipolar disorder. That isn't my burden. That isn't my fault.

Chapter 20

MAY 23, 2004
CINCINNATI, OHIO

Jessica's teachers came to her graduation party en masse. As did our family's church friends, neighborhood friends, and my parent's colleagues. And then there was family—our brother, Ben, came back from Providence; aunts and uncles and cousins traveled from all over the Midwest; and even my grandpa, the judge, flew down from St. Paul, Minnesota. Everywhere I looked, I saw someone who had played an important role in my life.

How many of them knew? How many of them had heard about the events of the past two months?

My palms sweated and my heart raced as I wandered through the party. I tried to avoid eye contact, and when that failed, I forced a smile and nodded, hoping to avoid conversation.

It was hopeless. These weren't distant acquaintances; these were people who loved me and wanted to connect. When I couldn't avoid conversations, I discovered my fears were warranted. When they asked, "How are you?" they asked with heightened concern, as if they knew the answer couldn't be, "I'm fine."

They knew. They all knew.

This was Jessica's party, but I could tell many of the guests were also here to check on me. There was a shadow side to the celebration, which my sister—who is ever so perceptive—surely sensed.

After a few awkward attempts at conversation, I sought out a hiding place. I slipped out the front door and collapsed into a wicker chair on our porch, the same spot where Jessica's eyes had told me her truth. Hiding from others was new to me and I wasn't very good at it. It wasn't long before my Aunt Margaret and Uncle Mike found me there. They sat down and asked me how I was doing.

Away from the hubbub of the party, I felt a bit safer and told them the truth. "I'm not well."

They rubbed my back gently, told me they had been praying for me, and handed me a small gift. It was a framed poem called *Footprints* about God carrying a man through his times of trial and suffering. I thanked Mike and Margaret for the gift, and they walked away. Later that day I placed it on my desk, where it remained—and over the years, I would look at it repeatedly and hope it was true.

I went back inside and walked among the guests—they were as cheerful and celebratory as I was dark and numb. I slipped through the crowd, feeling obligated to be there but trying to be invisible. When I reached another point of exhaustion, I escaped to the solarium.

The television was on, with athletes running around on the screen, and I sat on the couch and stared at them without watching. It was just me, and I hoped no one else would come in. But after a few minutes, my grandfather shuffled in—cane in hand, wearing a suit as he always did—and sat down next to me.

Grandpa Archie Gingold was beloved by almost everyone who knew him. He served as a Minnesota judge for decades, first in the St. Paul municipal courts and then on the Ramsey County district bench, where he spent eighteen years in the juvenile court. Wednesdays were his favorite days when he finalized adoptions. He would send his clerks out to buy cakes and turn his courtroom into a celebration.

Grandpa liked a good deal. He stocked up on essentials when they went on sale. When I was a teenager, he ran out of aftershave. He took my dad on an expedition around St. Paul to find the same brand, only to discover that it had been off the market for ten years—his supply had lasted that long.

Grandpa inherited some commercial properties from his father and acquired some of his own. He used the rents and his savings on aftershave to help his loved ones. Through generous annual gifts, he gave each of his grandchildren the opportunity to start their adult lives with a great education and without massive debt hanging over their heads.

His trip to Cincinnati for Jessica's graduation marked a milestone. She was his youngest grandchild. He was ninety-five years old and had attended all eight of his grandchildren's high school graduations.

When Grandpa sat next to me in the solarium, I was lost in my thoughts and lost in a house full of people. I felt like running but had no idea which direction to go. Grandpa and I hadn't spoken about my manic episode or hospitalization. I had no idea what my mother had told him, but I figured he had come in because he was tired of being on his feet in a crowded house.

I sank into the soft blue couch, with my feet glued to the floor, my arms at my sides, and my hands flat against the seat cushions. For a few minutes, we just sat there next to each other, staring at the television.

Then, without saying a word or looking away from the television, my grandpa reached over and placed his hand on top of mine. He wrapped his fingers under my palm. Immediately my eyes welled with tears as he gently squeezed.

His hands were polished and smooth, and he slowly ran his thumb across my fingers, rising and falling along the contours of my knuckles. Then his hand went still, just resting on top of mine. At first, his hand was cool—his elderly heart doing what it could to pump blood to the tips of his fingers. But, as it rested on top of mine, it grew warm. It was like I had slipped under a comforter on a cold winter night.

He didn't say a word; he just held me.

Chapter 21

JANUARY 18, 2023
St. Paul, Minnesota

O nly six of us have braved the subzero temperatures to come to the support group. Usually, the majority of the people who attend these meetings live with anxiety or depression rather than bipolar disorder. Tonight, though, four of the six people have bipolar disorder, and for once we are in the majority.

After our brief check-ins, sharing our names, diagnoses, and a few words about our weeks, the facilitator says, "Well, this is unusual."

We smile, all knowing that those with bipolar disorder are usually in the minority.

"Why don't we focus on our folks with bipolar disorder tonight."

She has depression, and she turns to the other group member who lives with that illness. "That okay with you?"

He smiles and nods.

The facilitator looks at me.

"Adam, why don't you start."

I take a deep breath and begin. They've heard it before, but I begin with my love for Montessori education and how heartbreaking it was to leave my lead teacher job after only a month.

I look around the circle and am encouraged by all the sympathetic eyes. I report that, on Friday, I was called in to sub at the school that I have been subbing at for a couple months. It was a great day, my first day as a sub during which I felt fully present.

Then I tell them about my therapist and how we've taken an unexpected deep dive into the first two years of my life with bipolar disorder. The manic episode, my hospitalization, my acceptance of my diagnosis, the long depression that followed, and my recovery.

I tell them about reconnecting with Patrick and how meaningful that is. I describe the awkwardness of spending so much time thinking about a chapter of my past while living with a wife and daughter who weren't a part of it.

A woman chimes in. "What you are doing is so important."

"Thank you," I say. "That's how I feel, but sometimes it's hard to talk about it. When people ask what you do, it's easier to say, 'I'm a teacher' than to say, 'I'm really deep in therapy.'"

Everyone chuckles.

Among these kindred spirits, a wave of gratitude sweeps over me. Not everyone gets this chance to take a break from work and from life and spend four months in the deep recesses of memory—dissecting a time of trauma and transformation and making sense of unwelcome events never successfully forgotten.

As other members of the group ask questions about my therapy, I realize it takes a certain courage to journey into the past and that, at times, my courage has faltered. I tell them that just a few weeks ago, I almost took a part-time job and got back to just moving on. But I didn't. I listened to an impulse that told me dealing with my past would lead to a better future.

I look around the room into the eyes of each person. The last thing I share lights up every face.

"I'm beginning to feel more whole."

Chapter 22

MAY–SEPTEMBER 2004
CINCINNATI, OHIO

When I got home from Jessica's graduation party, I brushed my teeth and shook a Zyprexa out of its bottle. I felt miserable. I had never been such a downer at a party. Instead of making people laugh, I was a subject of concern. Worse yet, the concern was warranted. Something was wrong with me. I had never felt this way before. The feeling was so new I couldn't even describe it. It was so uncomfortable and raw. It didn't feel natural, and it didn't feel right. I wasn't me.

I looked at the pill in my hand and remembered the first time I took Zyprexa. I was strapped down, with the nurses and doctors trying to convince me to take pills. I spat them out, then finally relented and swallowed. Becoming medicated wasn't a choice, not a real one.

The medications were powerful. I could feel it. Depakote, a mood stabilizer, came in pills the size of almonds, and I was supposed to swallow three. Zyprexa, an antipsychotic medication, was smaller but its effects were more dramatic— it slowed my body and deadened my spirit.

The meds were dragging me down. My thinking was foggy; my body was sluggish; and my voice slurred at times. I felt like a zombie. How much of what I was feeling was caused by the medications versus a mental illness?

I made a decision. The only way to know if something was really wrong with me was to stop taking my medications and see what happened. I returned the Zyprexa to its bottle.

As the days passed, a medication-induced fog lifted, and I could think clearly again. My mind was crisp; life was easier; and I had my old energy back. My doubts faded. I could trust myself. This was all a misunderstanding. A stress-induced break from normality. A one-time thing. I wasn't bipolar.

Two weeks later, I hadn't told anyone I went off my meds, and I was standing in my apartment talking to Kristin. Something I said or something I did, which I can't remember now, alarmed her. She saw a flash of the person I had become during my manic episode. And then I told her I had gone off my meds. Her eyes hardened. Her jaw clenched. She told me my manic episode was extremely hard on her and she couldn't go through that again.

She turned toward the door.

Life without her hit me. She was the last person I felt completely safe with. She still held me and listened to me. A wave of loneliness swept over me, and I knew it was self-induced. The behavior that had just alarmed her wasn't caused by my medications; it was caused by the mental illness the medications were designed to treat—I was going manic again. I had my answer.

"Wait," I said.

Kristin paused at the door.

"I'll go back on my medications."

She looked at me. Her body relaxed. She stayed.

My mania didn't fall off a cliff. Going off my meds gave it a little bump. Through the early summer, I still had bursts of energy, with moments when I felt fully alive and could socialize and be active. But by the middle of July, three months after my manic episode climaxed, it was over. I had come back down, and I kept on sinking.

My new apartment complex had a small swimming pool in the middle of the parking lot. Each day, I lounged poolside, swam a bit, and escaped my gloom through the magic of books. When a retired resident entered the pool area and disrupted my solitude, I hurried back up to my apartment, crawled into bed, and reopened my fantasy novels. Each afternoon, I got out of bed and walked to the neighborhood business district for a beer at Arlin's—almost always empty at that hour.

My big accomplishments of the summer were finishing the semester of classes disrupted by my hospitalization—taking one exam and writing a fourteen-page research paper—and taking a one-credit class at the zoo called Zoos as Classrooms. I needed one more semester of classes to graduate, but I knew my mind was dull—a result of my heavy doses of Zyprexa and Depakote and my near-constant thoughts of my illness—so I took precautions. I dropped my international affairs major, deciding to work toward a general liberal arts degree instead. Rather than take 300-level courses like International Political Economy and Post-Colonial Politics, I took classes in drawing, dance and movement—courses that didn't require high-level cognitive functioning.

But when classes started, so did the reality of returning to the scene of my manic episode. Every day, I walked past the apartment building where Kristin had lived, triggering memories of the scared look on her roommate's face as I stormed in and out of their apartment. The *Newswire* office was right in the middle of campus, and every time I saw it, I felt the intensity of my furor as I berated the editor. Memories of my manic episode haunted me whenever I wasn't in class, so I looked for places to hide.

At first, I hid in the student center, curled into an armchair on the second floor in the corner of the tower lounge. I closed my eyes and hoped to be left alone.

Then one day I heard what I had dreaded. "Adam!"

I opened my eyes and found an international student standing in front of me, a friend of a friend. He tried to strike up a conversation, and I attempted to muster the social skills to follow along, but all I wanted was to close my eyes and disappear. Soon, my one-word responses and lack of reciprocal questions brought the conversation to a close and he wandered away.

I exhaled. With my mouth dry and my muscles limp, I looked around at students wandering by and knew I needed a better place to wait for my next class. I left the lounge and walked to the library. On the second floor, in the middle of the stacks, I found a desk with cubicle walls. I crossed my arms on the desk and laid my head down, obscuring my face so no one would recognize me.

Soon, I heard footsteps and then a backpack hitting a desktop. The sound of a zipper and books being removed. I sneaked a look around the side of my desk, and sure enough, a student was sitting down to study at the desk in front of me.

I didn't know him, but what if he tried to talk to me? I didn't have the energy to engage in another conversation.

My forehead throbbed; my hands began to tremble; and my eyes began to water. As my heart raced, I unzipped my backpack and removed my bottle of Ativan. I walked to a water fountain, popped a pill in my mouth, took a swig of water, swallowed, and returned to my desk. After burying my head in my arms again, I waited to be numbed by the antianxiety pill. Eventually, my arms tingled, and my mind floated for a bit.

But soon, another student walked between the stacks, passed within inches of my desk, and sat at the desk behind me. Now I was surrounded. My heart rate picked up again. I clenched my entire body as I tried to hold it together.

It wasn't working. One pill was not enough.

I took another out of the bottle and returned to the water fountain. With twice the dose of Ativan entering my bloodstream, I sat at my desk, with my head still buried, and prayed the nausea in my gut would subside.

"Please, God," I whispered.

I felt myself breaking. I was about to crack open and sob, as I did in my apartment nearly every night.

No. Not here. Not now.

I grabbed my backpack and rushed out of the library.

Autumn wind stung my face as I hurried toward my car in the commuter parking lot. I collapsed into the driver's seat, reclined as far as possible, and closed my eyes. The tension that had grown over the last hour began to fade. When I opened my eyes and saw the blank fabric above me and the dark dome light, I felt a measure of peace. I had found a safe place to hide.

Two weeks later, I was back in the commuter parking lot, reclined as far as possible, but it was no longer a safe place to hide. The pain of returning to Xavier had found me even there.

I wanted to quit. My body was rigid, and my head felt crushed. My hand rested on my pocket, feeling my keys. A large part of me wanted to start the car and drive back to my apartment and never return to this place. Never.

The memories of my manic episode still ran through my head, but other memories had joined them, and they were almost more painful.

I remembered my life before my manic episode when I would sit in the front row of classes and shoot my hand in the air and when I thought deeply about comparative governance and international justice. I remembered who I had been before. And then I had to face who I had become—a ghost trying not to be seen.

For years to come, when I thought of my college years, I remembered the ghost I became and little else.

Chapter 23

SEPTEMBER– NOVEMBER 2004

CINCINNATI, OHIO

The freezer aisle beckoned with novelties.

I inched along, pushing a grocery cart containing a few apples, cereal, and milk—nothing that required preparation. In my depleted state, the chores of cooking and dishes felt unmanageable.

I had bought a couple of microwave dinners and some frozen chicken pot pies the week before. After warming my first frozen meal, I knew I was on to something. Microwave dinners didn't require cooking. They only required utensils, which I could find the energy to clean. They were apportioned, so there was no need to worry about serving sizes—they were sort of like going on a diet. That's how I thought of it—a microwave dinner diet.

They even sounded nutritious: Lean Cuisine, Healthy Choice, Smart Ones. At a minimum, frozen meals had to be healthier than fast food, which had dominated my diet since I had returned to Xavier a few weeks earlier.

I didn't know much about frozen cuisine. The only thing I knew was that I needed a lot of meals.

It was a struggle just to leave my apartment and be

in public. Buying several weeks' worth of food meant I didn't have to do it as often. I was in my own world as I filled my cart, designing my own diet, accommodating my need to just eat, not to cook or clean. I felt a rush of pride, and, for a moment, I was having fun. There was so much freedom in the freezer aisle, a vast expanse of options I had never considered before. It was like exploring a foreign country filled with easy delights—gifts I could unwrap every night. I felt like a child on Christmas morning, surveying a mountain of possibilities. I filled my grocery cart with pleasure.

As I wheeled my treasures to the checkout line, though, my positive energy drained away. I saw my cart as others might. It didn't look adventurous or fun—it just looked sad.

I avoided eye contact with the cashier as I loaded the dozens of frozen items onto the conveyor belt. My hands shook; my heart quickened; and my speech dried up. I watched the cashier swipe pot pie after pot pie and Lean Cuisine after Smart One. My palms sweated as I fumbled with my wallet.

What if the cashier said, "Wow, you really don't like to cook, do you?"

I could have simply said, "Yup, you got that right."

But that would have been a lie. I did like to cook. When I was a high schooler, I invented a dish made of hotdogs, onions, green peppers, and crushed red pepper flakes. I chopped everything up, sauteed it in butter, and then carefully scooped it all into two hot dog buns propped wide open. My taste buds met the savory rich hot dog first, then the spicy kick of the red pepper. It was good, but my pride made it taste better: I was a teenager. I cooked with vegetables. I was awesome.

I could have also told the cashier that I didn't have time to cook.

Another lie. I had plenty of time to cook. I spent hours lying around my apartment every day doing nothing at all, except watching television.

I could have also said, "I don't feel like cooking," and that would have been closer to the truth.

But the absolute truth of the matter—the truth I didn't want to face and the truth I certainly didn't want to share with anyone—was that I simply couldn't cook. It was impossible. The weight of my memories and my plunge into depression had flattened me to my bed. I was doing what I could to survive.

After paying, I loaded the groceries into my car, drove the few blocks to my apartment, and lugged them up the steps. My armpits and lower back were damp and rank from anxious sweat. I crammed all the food into the freezer, shut the door, and took a deep breath.

As the days passed, and my freezer's contents dwindled, I made many discoveries about frozen meals. There was the cardboard packaging with a metallic sheen that makes microwave pizza crispy instead of soggy. I slowly improved my peel—attempting to get the entire plastic cover off the compartmentalized food tray in one clean swipe. If I failed, slivers of clear plastic flopped into the puddles of gravy, and I had to fish them out and tear them off. The slivers sucked.

I learned not to judge a meal by its pre-microwave appearance—of course, chicken in peanut sauce doesn't look good frozen. I also learned not to judge a meal based on its post-microwave appearance—just stir the pools of liquid into the mashed potatoes and they taste fine.

There were setbacks. Some dishes were terrible, usually the ones that tried to be healthy—like a grilled fish filet with a side of rice and steamed vegetables. The fish, rice, and vegetables all tasted like hot water. Chewing the fish made my jaw bounce.

Meals with gravy or some sort of sauce were much safer. They, at least, had flavor.

And I learned that if a meal was truly awful, I always had a stash of Banquet chicken pot pies on hand—at one dollar each, they were a cheap insurance policy.

Perhaps the best thing about frozen meals was that they were easy to eat in front of the TV.

My TV screen was a mere thirteen inches. It sat on an end table. Directly in front of it, on the floor, was a twin-size futon mattress, with a backrest pillow at the head. When I lay on the futon, six inches off the ground, my toes touched the end table. My body was almost connected to the TV. At times, it felt like my survival was tied to it as well.

Television hadn't been a part of my life before my manic episode. But the summer after, I got cable. When the cable man left and I first flipped through all the channels, my body relaxed. The television embraced me, swallowed my attention, and welcomed me into worlds so far from my own.

If I was home, my television was likely on. In the mornings, I caught a few minutes before heading to my classes. In the afternoons, I bounced between my shows and my homework. Dinner was in front of the TV. And late into the night, the screen lit up my face, except when I stepped out on my balcony to smoke.

There were two things I watched that stretched on hour after hour, sucking me into a rhythm, and automating my focus.

On TNT, *Law & Order* began with a crime. Then there was an investigation. Then the twist. Then the district attorney had to choose whether to prosecute. Then they either got the guy or not. Then the theme song. Repeat. To this day, I can hear the theme song picking back up, episode after episode after episode.

On ESPN2, I got to know all the world's most talented poker players. Night after night, I would watch Texas Hold'em tournaments. The dealer flicked out the cards all the way around, and the players bent up the corner of their cards so a little camera could show me what they had. The dealer flipped over three cards in the middle, then another, and then another, with the players betting all along. The tension built, and then someone raked in the pot. Hand after hand after hand.

As the crimes were solved, and the cards were played, I grew numb, completely siphoned away from my feelings, and time slipped by unnoticed. It was a reprieve from my incessant thoughts of my manic episode and the devastating dread that depression had thrust upon me.

During every smoke break or dash to the bathroom, the television released its hold on me, and depression clamped down. My heart started racing; my hands shook and my mind thumped. A hammer began pounding me from head to toe, blow after blow. I couldn't dodge it, and the pain just mounted with each strike. The shift from the screen to the world was so difficult that, as soon as possible, I would scurry back, collapse onto my futon, and get sucked back into my television daze, where the pain disappeared. The world disappeared. I disappeared.

My television dependency only grew as my last semester of college proceeded. When my parents asked what I would like for a graduation present, I immediately answered: a new TV. Kristin went with me to buy it. We walked the aisles of Circuit City looking at TV after TV. They started small and cheap and got progressively bigger and more expensive. Since my parents were paying, I settled on a $400 twenty-seven-inch monster of a television. It was so deep I could barely fit my arms around it.

I hauled it up the three flights of stairs to my apartment and set it on the end table in front of my futon. The new television was twice as large as my last one, and it blanketed me in light. The screen encompassed me. It numbed my pain. The escape was just as complete, and far easier, than a Caribbean vacation. It was just a button-press away. Fifteen minutes in front of my new TV and I was in love.

Chapter 24

NOVEMBER–DECEMBER 2004

CINCINNATI, OHIO

D r. Gupta, my psychiatrist, looked at me from behind his ornate wooden desk. I slumped in a stiff armchair, looking down at the floor. His question lingered in the air—ever the first question of my appointments.

"How are you feeling?"

Oh, man. How was I feeling? The same as always. Exactly like last time. What did he want me to say?

What could I say beyond the usual? I didn't know. I didn't have the energy. I didn't really care. Nothing good came of those appointments, so why try?

"I feel shitty."

Of course, that wasn't enough for him. His questions came at me like a tsunami.

How would I describe my moods? My motivation? My energy levels? He wanted to know about my diet, my sleep, and my exercise. He asked about my anxiety level and my morning nausea.

I had no idea what to say.

Up until my diagnosis, I had always just lived. I hadn't

thought about any of those things. I certainly hadn't described them to anyone in detail.

But Dr. Gupta looked at me with expectant eyes and a pen poised above a notepad. I stammered out some words, not at all sure how accurate or descriptive they were. Then fell silent, feeling unqualified for the job of being mentally ill.

Dr. Gupta raised his eyebrows and named a medication that was meaningless to me, an amount that was either more or less, some side effects I should look out for, and slid a prescription across his desk.

I took the prescription to the pharmacy. A pharmacist gave me pills, which I took. Six weeks later, I was back in Dr. Gupta's office, saying the same thing: "I feel shitty."

If anything, I felt worse.

It was November, and my seven months on medications had been awful. The pills infuriated me.

In the hospital, I started on an antipsychotic and a mood stabilizer—Zyprexa and Depakote. Their job was to bring me under control and bring me down from the highest of highs, then hope they would keep me stable. I would have a steady mood and a functioning mind. They turned out to be 50 percent effective. They brought me down from mania, but then I sunk into a deep depression. From my perspective, they were a failure.

Dr. Gupta tinkered with my Zyprexa/Depakote regimen. He scaled back my dosages, hoping I would rise out of my stupor, but it didn't work.

With every adjustment, he advised me it might take a couple weeks to have an effect. Three weeks later, my mood slumped further when I realized the anticipated effect wasn't coming.

Then Dr. Gupta introduced an antidepressant.

He approached Prozac as if it was the most powerful force in the world. We would build up the dosage slowly, he told me, careful not to send me sailing up into mania again. He gave me the prescription and advised me that it was a very low dose, and it might take weeks to feel an effect.

Nothing. It changed nothing.

He upped the dose. Then upped it again. But it had no effect. I felt as shitty as ever.

I began to dread my visits to Dr. Gupta. I hated the waiting room. I hated sitting across from him with his desk between us. I hated finding new ways to describe how bad I felt. I hated his questions. I hated that I hung on to his every word.

Most of all, I hated the hope that flared up within me every time I reached across his desk and grabbed a new prescription.

Three weeks after Dr. Gupta increased my Prozac dosage for the second time, I was watching TV, and during a commercial break, my gaze turned inward. I felt no different. Getting out of bed hadn't become any easier. Life continued to be almost unbearable. I was as depressed as ever. I closed my eyes as a whisp of hope evaporated. Another medication change wasn't helping. I got up from the futon and grabbed my pack of cigarettes.

It was a mild November night, so I didn't bother putting on a coat when I stepped through the sliding glass door onto my balcony and collapsed into the red rocking chair. The other chair—an orange velvet armchair—was empty. Kristin was with friends, and she was the only person who ever sat there.

The balcony had a concrete floor, red brick walls, and a wrought-iron railing. An overhang protected it from any rain. The view was a busy four-lane street. Even at one a.m., steady traffic streamed by. I could see the convenience store across the street was open from its neon sign. Between the road and my apartment was a steep grass embankment that bottomed out near the foot of my building, three stories below, where an asphalt pad, about ten feet wide, ran the length of the building.

I lit a cigarette—bought by the carton across the Ohio River in Kentucky, the cheapest brand I could find. There was no point spending a lot of money when I was just trying to kill myself.

I took a drag, felt the nicotine tingle through my body, blew the smoke out, and let my inner turmoil loose.

The scenes ran through my head. Over and over again, there I was, hitting my mother and getting strapped down in the hospital. The memories were vivid, coursing through me and living in my flesh.

The person in those memories was me, but I had no control over him and was afraid of him. For all I knew, one morning I could wake up and he would be back.

The lights from the convenience store blurred as my eyes lost their focus.

There were three messages I had received from the doctors, books, and websites about bipolar disorder: lower my expectations for life, prepare for a long difficult path, and realize it might be fatal—one in three attempt suicide, and one in ten succeed.

I thought about my dry heaves that morning when I got out of bed, the sad excuses I made when Kristin asked me to go out with her friends, and how distant I had become from my family and friends. Then I thought about the time before it all began.

My carefree high school days.

My life-changing experiences in Kenya.

The exhilarating college years.

I thought about all I had done, how I had lived, and who I was before…this.

And what was *this*?

Depression?

No. It was more like drowning.

Every moment I felt a persistent tug down into an abyss. As far as I could see toward the horizon, there was no sign of relief. There were moments when the pain was so bad that I had to hide—in my car, a bathroom, my apartment—and just remember how to breathe.

That pain was like nothing I had ever experienced. Nothing I had ever known could exist. It was in the pit of my stomach—a dull stabbing or a garden trowel scooping out my insides. It felt like I was being strangled, with my airway constricted to the size of a cocktail straw. That was how I had to live—all day, in every moment—and no one could tell, except me.

I was dying a lonely death.

With one cigarette drag left, I stood up, pressed my body against the railing, and looked straight down at the asphalt.

Are three stories high enough to kill me? Do I need to jump head-first?

I took the final drag. The smoke swirled in my lungs but didn't fill the emptiness within. I flicked the cigarette butt into the darkness, watched the ember fall and the sparks fly when it hit the asphalt below.

My hands clasped down on the railing as I rocked on

my feet. The incessant memories. The haunting thoughts. I was long past crying about it. I was just numb.

Hollow.

Done.

I hated life. I hated feeling that way. I hated being bipolar.

I took a deep breath of cool air. A knot cinched down on my heart. My face quivered. My jaw clenched. My eyes bore into the asphalt.

I envisioned myself jumping. I pictured my body falling. I felt my skull crushing. I wanted to do it.

I wanted to die.

I stood there for a long time and savored the option of death. It didn't frighten me. It beckoned me. I considered it, envisioned it, and planned it. For the first time that day, I wasn't hiding from the pain. I just surrendered. And it was a welcome release.

My knees buckled, and I fell back into the rocking chair.

I put another cigarette between my lips and lit it.

I closed my eyes. My heart rate slowed. A wave of relief swept over me, but as soon as it passed, a deep dread settled in my gut. I would have to live another day. The thought made me grimace.

"Oh, God," I whispered.

"Please."

———

Dr. Wittstein, the psychologist the hospital referred me to for talk therapy, worked from her home on a Clifton hillside.

When I first stepped through her door, fresh out of the hospital, I regarded her with suspicion—was she another person trying to convince me I was sick? I tested her, carefully weighing her answers, and looking skeptically into her eyes. I learned she wasn't there to tell me anything; she was there to listen, which was great because I had a lot to say.

When I began to explore the possibility I had a mental illness, she helped me understand what it meant. She calmed my fears. She assured me being bipolar wasn't the end of the world. That I could trust my mind again. While I might always carry a diagnosis, it didn't have to define me. I was still me. I listened to her and wanted to believe her, but in my gut, I wasn't sure.

Dr. Wittstein witnessed me fully accept I had bipolar disorder. I poured out all my big questions, received her answers, and slipped deep into the depths of depression.

On a cold December day, I went into Dr. Wittstein's house, sat down on her couch, and looked at her with frightened eyes.

"How are you, Adam?" she asked.

I opened my mouth to answer, but no words came out.

Nothing had changed since our previous week's session. I had never felt worse in my entire life, but I had been telling her this for months now.

I didn't feel like myself. I was losing hope. I saw no light at the end of the tunnel.

I looked at her with my mouth open, my cheeks twitching, and slowly shook my head from side to side.

What was life without a future? Without light? Without a self? Would it ever be possible to escape the memories that followed me everywhere?

Those were the questions I asked God on my balcony when I stood pressed against the wrought-iron railing.

Our sessions had grown quieter and quieter until there was silence interrupted by a few feeble whispers. Finally, I told Dr. Wittstein about the balcony.

The truth didn't come easily. It rose up like morning sickness, with painful heaves. For twenty minutes, I hunched on her couch trying to get through a sentence.

"Sometimes…"

I looked into her eyes, searching for mercy. But the truth needed to be spoken.

"Sometimes…I stand…"

I fell silent, into a state of uncontrollable grief. I shifted on the sofa, and the tiny movement took up all of my energy. I opened my mouth several times and leaned forward, only to have my chin slump down into my chest before I was finally able to release a few more words.

"Sometimes, I stand at my balcony…"

At this point, enough of my darkness had escaped that it shadowed the room—it hovered over us, and I was afraid to face it, so I kept my head down and spoke into my lap.

"Sometimes, I stand at my balcony, up against the railing…"

My eyes glazed over—I was on the balcony, pressed up against the railing. I could feel the wrought iron digging into my upper thighs—my heart thumping wildly, my mind lost in a thick fog, and my soul tired of asking questions of God.

"…and look down."

The peace of death settled over me. Tears flowed, coming from a place of suffering beyond myself. I was adrift. Soulless and lost. Sleeping away the day and emerging at night. Tomorrows were becoming less and less likely as I spent more time each night pressed up against the railing. I was tired of waking up.

On my therapist's couch, my conversation with God burst into the world. My life had become a struggle with death.

No one knew I was suicidal until that moment.

I looked up from my pants and into Dr. Wittstein's eyes. Her eyes were filled with concern, with mercy, and with love.

She pushed the tissue box across the coffee table and waited for me to dry my tears. She let the truth linger in the room for a while, adjusting to its freedom, stretching out from the cramped confines of my soul.

She watched me take a deep breath and shudder the last of my shudders. Then she spoke.

"Give it time, Adam, give it time."

Time.

Time.

Time.

We sat there in silence for the rest of our time together.

Time.

Time.

Time.

We spent many more sessions silently sitting together.

Time.

Time.

Time.

Together, we gave it time.

Time.

Time.

Time.

Alone, I gave it time.

Time.

Time.

Time.

And, with time, I got better.

Chapter 25

JANUARY 24, 2023
St. Paul, Minnesota

"Why didn't you jump?"

For some reason, when I brought up my suicidal thoughts, I wasn't expecting Dr. Fossum to ask about them.

But now she has. And for the first time since I moved out of my third-floor apartment seventeen years ago, I return to the core of that dark time.

A stream of platitudes flows through my mind. I still had a shred of hope. I didn't want to hurt my loved ones. I was too scared to jump. None of them ring true.

I tell Dr. Fossum about Dr. Wittstein's advice, to give it time. How I could choose between death and time. So, I chose the latter. But even that doesn't seem complete.

I shake my head. "I don't know."

We move on and discuss other topics, but I'm distracted by her earlier question. So I return to it.

"When I was alone on my balcony, I spoke with God about jumping. I always had a conversation going. I was never completely alone. I think I didn't jump because I still believed in something."

She asks a few follow-up questions, then says, "I think that time on your balcony was very important. During your depression, it seems that was when you were most alive. You were facing it. You were inside your body."

I think back to that horrible year, hiding in bed, in novels, in my car at school, and the endless hours in front of my TV. I hid from a lot of things. But I didn't hide from my suicidal thoughts.

Dr. Fossum's words mean something important. I'm sure of it. But even as I look at her and nod, I don't quite understand.

I'm on a walk when Dr. Fossum's words return to me.

How was I most alive when I was considering suicide?

As my feet fall one after the other, I allow myself to do something I haven't done since I moved out of that third-floor apartment: I return to my body when it was pressed up against the railing.

I feel the allure of the plunge, the surrender to depression's tug, and the only blessed moments of those days when I wasn't running and hiding from the pain. And then I understand Dr. Fossum's words.

Suicidality is a symptom of severe depression. The nights when I considered suicide, I was facing one of the hardest parts of living with my illness. Those nights were not a personal failure or a self-induced trauma. I was just miserably sick and that wasn't my fault.

I haven't told very many people I considered suicide. I've never known how to talk about it. Somehow, I got the message that suicidality is something to hide, something to be ashamed of.

But there is no reason to run from my memories of the nights I considered suicide. They were meaningful.

Throughout my worst depression, those were the moments I really faced my suffering. Those nights on my balcony were the truest part of my severe depression, when I was most in my body, grappling with the pain, and living my life as it was at that time.

My walk leads me to the Mississippi River—near the place where I took a picture of its frozen waters and texted it to Patrick. Except here there is a rocky outcropping and a drop of about forty feet to the riverbank strewn with boulders.

Ever since those nights on my balcony, when I have approached a ledge, I've felt an urge to jump, as if a phantom tug from my most depressed days still lingers in my muscles. My legs begin to wobble as I near a drop-off, my pulse quickens, and I sink low to the ground as I hastily retreat.

Standing about ten feet from the edge of the outcropping, my body feels different. It isn't shaky. My heartbeat is steady. I don't feel a tug. So, I creep forward until my toes are within a few inches of the rim.

I look down at the boulders and remember those many nights on my balcony looking down at the asphalt. I take a deep breath. My body's calm tells me that the memories have changed. They don't feel the same. Embracing them has somehow altered them. Instead of terrorizing me, the memories seem to have settled into my past, into an empty spot in my story, an important part of my story.

I'm not afraid. I feel no impulse to jump. My legs stand firm.

I've feared heights for so long now that it never occurred to me that I could someday stand at a ledge and feel as I do at this moment.

I feel safe.

Down to the marrow of my bones, for the first time since I was suicidal, I fully trust myself.

Chapter 26

DECEMBER 2004–
OCTOBER 2005

CINCINNATI, OHIO

Soon after my hospitalization, I started attending a bipolar support group. Some members had lived with bipolar disorder for many years. Others were young, like me, still trying to come to terms with their diagnosis.

A mental health professional facilitated the group, which met in a hospital. Many of the members were people who had recently been hospitalized. As a result, there was an absence of laughter and a plethora of traumatic stories. It may not have been an uplifting group, but it was one of the only places outside my therapist's office where I could talk about what was really going on in my mind. It was a refuge, and for that I was grateful.

Most weeks, when I arrived at the hospital, my parents were waiting for me at the hospital doors. While I met with my group, they met with a support group for families of people with bipolar disorder. Seeing them triggered waves of emotion—gratitude they showed up for me, anger for hospitalizing me, shame for how I had behaved during my manic episode, and the ever-present tug to hide from them and from everyone.

When I was finishing up college, the facilitator of the support group offered me a job at the Respite Center, a mental-health-crisis stabilization center, which she managed. I took the job and was scheduled to start soon after my finals.

When I turned in my last exam, completing the requirements for my degree, I didn't feel accomplished or proud of my achievement. I felt emaciated, as if I had survived a tortuous journey through a desolate landscape that I never wanted to see again—a place and time I just wanted to forget.

I didn't attend my college graduation ceremony. I didn't care if they mailed me my diploma. I just slipped away from Xavier University and had no desire to ever look back.

Starting work at the Respite Center was a relief. Spending forty hours a week surrounded by people with mental illnesses was comfortable. My job was to keep the residents safe and fed, and dole out their medications, all of which I could do, even in my depleted state. I worked the evening shift, from four p.m. to midnight, giving me an excuse for not having much of a social life. The job was a perfect fit.

My life fell into a predictable rhythm. For most of my days, I slept in, went to work, came home, watched TV, spent some time on my balcony, and repeated it the next day. For companionship, I had Kristin, who spent many nights at my apartment after I picked her up from her server job late at night. On the weekends, she would sometimes coax me out to bars with her friends—they had fun, while I forced a smile and willed myself not to run home early.

My work gave me energy at first—I enjoyed learning a new job and getting better at it. But within a month, most lessons were learned, and the shifts started blurring together.

During my first winter and spring with bipolar disorder, I had a job, my TV, frozen meals, and Kristin's companionship. My basic needs were met, but my inner self continued eroding. I needed a boost.

When my one-year lease expired at the end of May, I moved in with Kristin. We rented a second-floor apartment in an old building with high ceilings and ornate woodwork. The apartment had a balcony, but below it was a carpet of grass.

The absolute worst of my depression was behind me. I had adapted to a sadder life. Time had soothed the sting of my illness. But life with bipolar disorder still felt like a shadow of the life I had enjoyed without it. When I looked in the mirror, I saw a man who had survived but hadn't yet learned to thrive.

That summer, to earn extra income, I took a second job working three days a week for a landscaping company. I wanted to be outside, move my body, and get in better shape. But I had some trepidation because I was taking on far more than I had at any point since my diagnosis.

On Mondays, Wednesdays, and Fridays, between my two jobs, I worked fifteen-hour days. On Tuesdays and Thursdays, I only worked at the Respite Center, so I had those mornings to sleep in and recover. It was demanding, but at the end of each day, I came home feeling accomplished.

Early one morning, our work crew arrived in a huge suburban yard with a garden bed running along the entire front of a McMansion. The bed was in bad shape. It was an ugly design to begin with, and grass had crept underneath the bushes further marring its appearance.

My boss walked a curving path through the yard a few feet out from the bushes and asked who was willing to carve the edge. It was a beast of a job, about as demanding as a suburban edging job can be. I volunteered.

A properly landscaped yard needs clean edges. Some machines can cut edges along sidewalks or flower beds, but there is also an edging spade—a flat shovel with a waist-high D-grip handle. It was the only edging tool we had, so I grabbed it and walked to one end of the garden bed.

After about fifteen minutes, I got into a smooth rhythm, placing the shovel, stepping it down a few inches, lifting it up to loosen the dirt, and placing it again, moving down the length of the new bed. Once I reached the end, I looked back at my work—a smooth undulating outline cutting through the yard. Pleased, I reversed course, holding my edging spade nearly parallel to the ground. I thrust it forward, scraping away the top two inches of earth and its clingy grass between the line I had cut and the bushes.

It took the entire morning. When I finished, I looked back at the bed. A few hours earlier, it had been a weedy mess. Now, a clean edge defined a flowing bed—a serene sight. And I had created it. As we packed up for lunch, my boss came over to admire my work.

"Damn, Adam, that's a good edge."

I became the go-to guy for edges. When possible, they saved the edges for the days I worked. For the first time in over a year, I was the best at something, and I knew it. I was The Edging Man.

During that summer, my confidence grew. Since finish-ing school, I had slept through most mornings, sometimes getting out of bed only a couple hours before my shift at the Respite Center started at four p.m. But now, I was working from seven thirty a.m. to midnight, with only a short break between jobs. It was an intense schedule, but it gave me pride. For the first time in a long time, I felt capable of accomplishing hard things. I felt strong.

As summer waned and the landscaping work dried up, I found myself asking a new question.

Instead of "Do I want to live?" I asked, "What do I want to do with my life?"

Maybe, I thought, *I want to be a psychologist.*

The large lecture hall at the University of Cincinnati was filled with undergrads, and I wondered why they were there. Perhaps they were majoring or minoring in psychology or fascinated by the way the mind operated. Or maybe they were learning to live with a mental illness like me and thought they could help others going through something similar.

I sat through the prerequisite classes for a graduate psychology degree—classes I didn't take during my own undergraduate education—one of dozens, if not hundreds, of anonymous students.

I imagined myself getting a PhD. I would do clinical work, sit down with people struggling as I was, talk them through it, and let them know it was okay. All too quickly, that fantasy collided with reality.

Within a few weeks, that much focus on mental illness became overwhelming. Each day, I woke up and took my medicine, and biked to my psychology classes. Then I rushed to my job at the Respite Center dealing with people in a mental health crisis. In my free time, I saw my psychologist and psychiatrist to deal with my illness.

My life became consumed with mental illness.

Not long into the semester—after reviewing my classes' syllabi and completing a few reading assignments—I realized how difficult it would be to get from where I was to a PhD.

The daily homework piled up. The reading assignments were long and barely held my attention. I admitted to myself I wasn't there to help others so much as to understand myself. My motivation slipped.

It was a large cognitive leap from edging a garden to studying for a graduate degree. I made it to midterms but no further. I dropped out.

Instead of sitting in lecture halls, I returned to my television, watching old episodes of *Columbo*, waiting for my shift at the Respite Center, and feeling lost once again. The burst of energy and motivation I had received from landscaping and returning to school slipped away. I fell into a funk. I wanted to have direction, purpose, and excitement, but I had forgotten how to find it, and depression came nipping at my heels.

The only thing notable on my calendar for the rest of the year was two months away—an upcoming family vacation to Brazil between Christmas and New Year's.

―――

Just after I dropped my classes, I had an appointment with Dr. Gupta. I told him about dropping out of school and how I felt my depression growing. He suggested I start on a drug called Lamictal.

As Dr. Gupta slid an orange and blue starter pack across his desk, he told me that Lamictal was new, so there wasn't much known about it, but it seemed effective at treating bipolar depression. After no success with Depakote or antidepressants, it was hard to be optimistic about a new medication. It didn't help that the initial doses were the size of the gravel in the bottom of a fish tank—how could the tiny things have any effect?

And yet, despite my doubts, I couldn't suppress the sliver of hope I always felt as I left my psychiatrist's office with a new prescription.

Week by week, as the dose slowly increased, to my surprise, my mood improved. The shift wasn't dramatic, but it was noticeable. The painful pangs of depression became less frequent. I had more energy. Every part of life was just a little bit easier. The darkening mood I had felt building subsided.

At the end of the first month, for the first time in eighteen months, when I sat down across from Dr. Gupta who asked me how I was feeling, I didn't say, "Shitty."

Instead, I said, "Pretty good."

The relief from depression's persistent tug was a welcome change. But over the previous eighteen months, I had established new habits, a new way of life, and even a new way of thinking about myself. As Lamictal freed my moods from the grip of depression, my self-image was still trapped in a pill bottle.

I had become so used to being shrouded by depression, that when the veil lifted, I wasn't sure what to do. I had forgotten how to be healthy. My social life, diet, and physical fitness had all atrophied due to my depression. My job was a result of attending the support group, and it rarely challenged me. Almost everything about my life came back to my illness. Lamictal improved my mood, but only I could improve my life.

Chapter 27

JANUARY 27, 2023
St. Paul, Minnesota

I've been on Lamictal for the last seventeen years. Combined with other medications, therapies, and self-monitoring, I haven't experienced another manic or depressive episode as severe as my first. What I have experienced more regularly is hypomania, which is what I'm feeling tonight.

My fingers are wrinkled from the bath, but I linger in the warm water. A scented candle casts a warm glow on the tile walls. My frenetic energy has calmed. This is a familiar ritual.

It's been about a week of uneven sleep. I've had to take Temazepam, my antianxiety drug, four times to get to sleep. I can't stop thinking about a long list of projects and decisions. All day I was on the move, from one task to another.

I told Meredith earlier: "I'm a bit hypomanic. Nothing to be concerned about, but I'm going to try and chill out tomorrow."

Nothing to be concerned about? Really? Am I really not concerned? This is new.

Since I met Meredith sixteen years ago, whenever I've felt this way and recognized it as hypomania—that revved-up state characterized by many of the same symptoms as mania, but not so severe that they impair my relationships or land me in the hospital—I've been concerned.

Fearing a full-blown manic episode is just a step away, I've taken immediate and decisive action: check off the urgent items on the to-do list, take a twenty-minute bath, fire up the TV, get my favorite snacks, secure a mindless novel, and veg out until my spirit settles. Withdraw from the world. Fend off any further movement toward mania. Do whatever it takes to regain my equilibrium.

The water laps against the bathtub walls as I shift position. A question formulates in my mind.

How does it feel to be hypomanic?

The question surprises me because I've never asked it before. In the past, fear consumed me at these moments, and I focused on where I might be headed rather than where I was.

I feel amped up but also somewhat exhausted. A bit dizzy, but also creative and productive.

In the last three days, I've taught myself how to lay tile and built a hearth extension for our fireplace—a project that could have easily dragged on for a week or more.

My thoughts are focused on tiny details and grand visions. House projects run through my mind step by step in a stream of consciousness.

When I open my mouth to speak, the words cascade one after another, a surge I find hard to stop. When a person gets my attention, I zero in on them and on what it is they really want. But getting my attention is hard, as my mind seems to focus at will—its will.

Hypomania isn't a bad feeling, but it's not a great one either. And it's confusing, because the line between normal mood swings and bipolar-induced ones isn't always clear.

The extreme mania and depression I experienced after my diagnosis were easy to identify. But everything in between can feel muddled, so much so that when I'm feeling off, I often call it a "roughening"—not a clinical term, but one that seems better suited to my murky reality than a definitive term like "hypomania."

Do I want to stay in this state a bit longer?

No. I want to get some sleep and get my equilibrium back, but I don't want to overact. There is nothing bad about being hypomanic. This isn't a failure. I don't need to dissect the last week, looking for triggers so I can try and avoid them in the future. I am bipolar. Sometimes this will happen, and that's okay.

Really, Adam? Do you really feel this way?

Yes. Really.

A tension I've felt ever since I came to terms with my diagnosis relaxes. An overbearing sense of responsibility evaporates. Eighteen years of trying to solve my illness, trying to achieve a perpetual state of perfect mental health—gone.

It's okay. You are okay just the way you are.

The espresso maker hums. A splash of milk, and I sit down to write. Phoenix and Meredith sleep as my fingers fly. Last night, I awoke at 2:00 a.m., then 4:00 a.m., and finally got up at 5:50 a.m. But I didn't have to take Temazepam to fall asleep, an improvement.

It's my fourth attempt at getting my experience down in writing. The first three times, spaced out over ten years, never felt complete and never felt good enough to share. This time though, it feels different; it feels right.

If this had been any time since my diagnosis up to this moment, a few nights of fitful sleep would wreck me with anxiety. I know very well that with bipolar disorder, rough sleep can lead to rough moods—and there is no better way to regulate my mood than to get quality sleep. After a week of cruddy sleep, I usually spend the whole day fretting about getting to sleep that night.

But, yesterday, I was hypomanic and still able to fall asleep without drugs. The day was extremely productive and filled with energy, but the long wind-down worked. The bath at six thirty p.m., a show, a book, and then bed.

Huh? Maybe I should try it again today. Ride this hypomanic energy, attack some projects, and then, when the day starts to wane, chill out and prepare my mind and my body for sleep, trusting I'll get enough to prevent full-blown mania.

Manage it; do not fear it. Dance; do not retreat. Breathe.

I hear Phoenix's door open upstairs and then her footsteps as she runs into our bedroom to cuddle with Meredith, as she does every morning.

Downstairs, in the kitchen, I get out the eggs and the English muffins and begin making breakfast. The toaster oven's element glows red. The butter in the skillet sizzles.

"Breakfast," I call up the stairs.

Meredith comes down first.

As she makes her morning latte, I tell her, "I slept better last night."

She looks up at me.

"I didn't have to take Temazepam. I'm still feeling hypomanic, but I'm just going to use that energy and stay busy today, and then chill out in the evening before bed."

She smiles.

"It worked yesterday," I say. "Maybe it will work again today."

She seems relaxed, with none of that tension I often see in her when I'm in a roughening. "Okay," she says with apparent calm. "Sounds good."

These episodes, for the entirety of our relationship, have been awkward, frightening, and often lacking in communication. I told her early on in our years together that, when I'm feeling off, I need to cancel everything, and crawl into bed with a book and a screen until the impending storm dissipates. This was hard for her—she wanted to do something to help. Snuggle me, make me food, talk. But all I want at those times is space; I want her to leave me alone. So now, she buys me 7-Up and cranberry juice, popcorn, and cheese and protects my peace. When I've been in a roughening, we've never had a conversation like this.

It feels good. It feels like growth.

The next day, I visit a chiropractor. I've been enduring neck pain for a couple weeks, so I finally made this appointment. It's my first time visiting her, and when I arrive, she takes me back to the treatment room. Then she asks me what I do.

"I'm a substitute teacher, and I'm working on a book."

"Oh," she says with a bounce. "What is the book about?"

"It's a memoir about living with bipolar disorder."

Her bounce settles and she says, seriously, "I'm sorry you have to live with that."

I've never gotten that response.

I normally try to fend off such expressions of sympathy, assuring people that I'm fine, know how to manage it, and am actually proud of how much I have achieved despite it.

But this time I say nothing and allow her words to penetrate.

That night, I'm back in the bath. The hypomania hasn't receded, and I'm second-guessing this new approach. Maybe I should just retreat and recover. Last night I slept terribly again, and I just want to settle, to sleep well, and to feel calm.

The longer I soak, the more the concerns of that moment dissipate, and a larger grief settles over me. It is a soul space I avoid, an admission I skirt, but it is also inescapably true. I do not want to be bipolar. I really don't.

Chapter 28

DECEMBER 24, 2004– JANUARY 1, 2005

BRAZIL

I had been anxious about our family trip to Brazil. Despite my progress, a year-and-a-half after my hospitalization, my confidence and vitality weren't back to their previous levels. Certainly not up to international-travel levels.

The trip began with a shock. As we drove away from the airport with the guide my mother had hired, we asked a few questions about the itinerary and began to suspect he didn't have one. By the end of our first day, we were sure of it—he was flying by the seat of his pants.

My family likes vacations packed with experiences, learning, and adventures. They want to know where, what, when, how, and why. They don't want to laze about at a fancy hotel pool on the outskirts of a bustling town—which was the guide's plan for our first two days in Manaus.

So, we fired our guide and set off on our own.

To plan a foreign vacation on the fly, we had to muster all our resources. My brother's long-term girlfriend, Katy, spoke Portuguese and became our communicator. My mom gave us guts, and my brother Ben's level head helped us stay calm. My dad mediated disputes while Jessica brought her empathy so we could emote. Our cousin Carrie set boundaries so we wouldn't take on too much. Kristin was new to international travel and gave us a sense of wonder—and I had to contribute something too.

Throughout our childhood, Jessica helped her friends distinguish between her brothers by describing Ben as "the hot one" and me as "the funny one." But during my long depression, I wasn't funny. I was sick.

I had disappeared from family life. I didn't read historical fiction with my dad. I didn't laugh at my mom's hilarity. I didn't play sports with Ben when he came to town. I wasn't the person my sister could call in tears. I was none of that. Years later, Jessica told me, "I lost my brother for a year."

But something happened in Brazil. When our family needed to pull together and make the best of an unfortunate situation—I rediscovered my humor.

Instead of looking for opportunities to pull back and sequester myself, I followed conversations, looking for opportunities to interject with a quip, especially when things were getting heated between the many opinionated people in our family. My humor diffused many disputes and brought levity to what could have been a tension-filled trip.

With my sense of humor, I was welcomed back to the family table as if I had never left.

The trail to the waterfall was a mile long. It had a gentle grade and was wide and well-packed. I figured I would be fine wearing flip-flops, a swimsuit, and a T-shirt. I had forgotten that with my family, the trail only begins where the wide, leisurely trail ends.

When everyone else followed the narrow side trail into the jungle, I didn't want to be left behind, so I scurried after them. I tried to keep up as they worked their way over large roots, around muddy pits, and under dense foliage. No one knew where the path led. It was unmarked, but that's why we were following it—my family had a thing for going to the end of the world.

Crawling through the jungle, I began to wonder if I too was, once again, capable of tackling uncharted territory. Yes, I was bipolar now and fifty pounds heavier than during our last family vacation. But there I was straddling large logs, squatting under branches, and leaping over mud puddles. As I stretched my leg over a downed tree, I heard it—my swimsuit splitting in the crotch, from waistline to waistline. I stopped, slumped, and watched my family disappear into the jungle ahead.

I turned back toward our van, but after just a few steps, the center anchor of my right flip-flop tore through the sole.

Barefoot and with a gaping hole in my swimsuit, I fought my way out of the jungle, covered in mud and defeated. I trudged back up the wide, leisurely trail. Trying to hold my swimsuit closed just drew more attention from the other tourists, but what else could I do? I felt an overwhelming urge to catch the next flight home and crawl back inside my carefully cultivated comfort zone.

———

The next day, we flew into Rio de Janeiro, rented cars, and drove up the coast to celebrate the New Year in a small beach town. Staying in a bed and breakfast directly on the beach, I could hear the waves crashing from my bedroom. And I had no swimsuit.

Brazilians like flesh. They take a minimalist approach at the beach. Women wear string bikinis that disappear between their butt cheeks. Men, not to be outdone, display their assets in tight swim briefs.

The beach shops catered to the local tastes in beachwear—not to American tourists. As I flipped through a stack of Speedos, heavier than I had ever been, the best I could hope for was to find something, anything, that fit. I found only one that might possibly fit—navy blue with two white stripes along the side.

I held it up and imagined putting it on, and the hilarity of the situation struck me.

If I wore this suit casually and confidently, as if it was tailor-made, I could shine. I could be the envy of my family. I could pretend to blend into the local beach scene—a ludicrous proposition given that I was a hairy beast in the country that gave us the Brazilian wax.

I imagined how good it would feel standing on the beach snugly tucked into a Speedo. My anxiety and fear gave way to the spirit of adventure.

I bought the navy-blue Speedo, and I was right—standing on the beach in it felt great, no matter how I appeared. I wore it with such style and grace my brother bought one too. He had never emulated me before.

Two days later, on New Year's Day, I walked out onto the beach alone and gazed at the Atlantic Ocean crashing on the white sand beach. A deep desire for change swept over me.

My life was stuck and had been for a long time. Bipolar disorder had control. It was time for that to change. It was time to move out from under the shadow of my illness. It was time for me to take charge and get healthy. When I got home, I told myself, I was going on a diet, getting in shape, getting a different job, perhaps internationally related, and quitting smoking.

I set lofty goals, especially considering my recent track record. But, for the first time since my diagnosis, I felt capable. I felt like living.

Chapter 29

FEBRUARY 3–6, 2023
CINCINNATI, OHIO, AND
HARBOR SPRINGS, MICHIGAN

As I exit the Cincinnati airport, Geoff pops out of his car and dances toward me with a big smile on his face. "Adam G!" he shouts, laughing.

We have a weekend of fun in front of us. For me, it's a much-needed escape from the intensity of therapy, the uneasiness of being unemployed, and not knowing my next move. I haven't felt like this since I dropped my psychology courses seventeen years ago. I even watched two episodes of *Columbo* last week.

I stay the night with Geoff's family, and the next morning we wake early, meet up with our friends Chuck and Dave, and hit the road—eight hours north to snowy Michigan.

The drive is awesome. We're in our forties now and we know stuff—experts, even, in many things—so our conversations are detailed and deep. We discuss the intricacies of artificial intelligence, the workings of cryptocurrency, the Columbian exchange, bipolar disorder, parenting, and marriage. And we laugh, holding fast to the immature humor of our adolescence.

How could jokes about my infatuation with Chuck's older sister ever not be funny? Sure, she's married and has kids now. But I'm convinced she thinks of me as the one who got away—a fantasy my friends have been laughing about for twenty-five years.

It's dark when we arrive at our rented condominium in the Michigan countryside. We eat pizza and play a round of euchre. With our heavy drinking days behind us, we sip peppermint tea and then, one by one, head up to bed. I sleep poorly again, as I did at Geoff's the night before, but wake up with the pent-up energy of needing time with old friends.

We ski through the morning, then find a table at a mountaintop chalet to eat our packed lunch. At a nearby table, a large family dressed in American flag ski suits, with two-way radio speakers clipped to their shoulders, sits together. Even though they're right next to each other, they still speak through their radios, filling the air with occasional crackles as the radios go on and off. I watch them for a while but then turn my gaze inward.

Something is off. My mood feels shaky. As I take the final bites of my peanut butter and jelly sandwich, my energy leaves me. My body feels heavy. My hope was that the food would give me a boost, but it seems to be having the opposite effect.

My friends munch away, observing the colorful crowd, chuckling as their conversation flows. But I'm quiet. I'm listening to myself.

Two nights of poor sleep. Two days of excitement. And my equilibrium is thrown.

This is a familiar conundrum—after a few days into a highly anticipated trip, I feel my mood shift. The break in routine, the unfamiliar beds, the overstuffed pillows, the invigorating newness of the moment. Sleep becomes elusive, and I feel a roughening—my mind racing about; my body restless, tired, and wired at the same time; a distance forming between me and the people around me; and the slumping acceptance that life is a bit harder for me.

In the past, I've fought it and struggled to be there for everything, silently pushing myself to my limits, and then frantically retreating to regain my balance.

Today is different. The struggle has left me.

My friends want to ski some more after lunch, go back to the condo for dinner, and then return to the slopes for night skiing. My options are clear in my mind. I see the three ways the day could play out.

I could stifle my unease and stick with the guys and tag along for everything, growing quieter as my inner focus turns to my mental health. I would be with them physically but not in the ways that count.

Or I could punt the decision to later—no need to decide on night skiing until I see how I feel after dinner. But I already know that if I don't decide now, I'll be thinking about the choice until it's made.

Or I could follow a path that returns me to health, so I can be with my friends in the ways that really matter.

As my friends finish their lunches, I tell them I'm not feeling great. I'm tired and haven't been sleeping well, and my bipolar disorder is flaring a bit. I tell them I'm going to stay in the chalet while they ski that afternoon, and that after dinner, I'm going to chill out and take a bath rather than go night skiing.

They understand. They say they'll just do a few runs, then we can head back to the condo. It isn't a big deal. It really isn't. Not for them. And, for once, not for me.

They put their ski gear back on and push off down the mountain. From where I sit, looking out the window, I can see the top of the chairlift. Each time they return to the top of the mountain, they ski past me and make funny faces through the window. I smile at them and am so happy to be where I am, with them, as myself.

____

My night at the condo rejuvenates me. The next day, we ski some more and then drive back to Cincinnati. Even with my mental health roughening, the getaway was just what I had hoped for. But the following morning is the moment of the trip I've been anticipating the most.

I'm sitting in a Cincinnati café, a few hours before my flight back to St. Paul, sipping a cup of coffee. Just as I take the last sip, my phone lights up.

"I'm here."

I look up and survey the café.

Did Patrick slip in without me noticing?

No, I don't see him. Then, out the window, I see movement, and there he is. Patrick. Getting out of his car.

He sees me through the window and his rich black face breaks open into a glistening smile. His smile. The smile I've loved since the day I met him. The smile I haven't seen for eighteen years.

My face returns the welcome as I rise from my seat to meet him at the door. We throw our arms around each other in a long and strong embrace. We utter greetings with our cheeks touching.

A waiter fills his coffee cup. Patrick doesn't even look at the menu, just orders what I order. And we listen to each other. No interrupting. No finishing of each other's sentences. Just long-delayed confessions of the heart. We've both carried the emptiness of each other's absence but in vastly different ways.

He stayed in Cincinnati, surrounded by our friends, but traveled alone instead of with me by his side. And for eighteen years, the questions never ceased.

"Where is Adam these days? What is he doing?"

For eighteen years, he hasn't had an answer. He doesn't understand why I withdrew or why our relationship faded. My absence left a hole in his life that everyone could see.

I tell him why I disappeared. First into the hospital, as he knows, then into a deep depression and the slow climb out of it, and then off to Washington, DC, to begin anew. But his absence traveled with me. There was also a hole in my life, but no one around me knew him or how much I loved him. I carried his absence quietly but always.

We don't move on from the topic. For two hours, we discuss our friendship, our feelings, our place in each other's lives, and in each other's story. When it comes time for me to go to the airport, he offers to drive me.

When we pull up at the airport departures, he gets out of the car and opens the hatch. He puts my suitcase on the ground as I put my backpack on. We face each other and once again envelop each other in our arms.

"I love you, Adam," Patrick says into my ear.

"I love you too," I reply.

I give him a strong squeeze, pull away, and turn to walk into the airport. As I near the door, I look back at his car and see he is already back in the driver's seat but I stand there a moment, just existing.

When I finally walk through the sliding doors into the terminal, I feel a deep sense of peace. It is an entirely new feeling—like every shattered piece of my soul has finally aligned.

Chapter 30

JANUARY–APRIL 2006

CINCINNATI, OHIO

A week after returning from Brazil, I settled into a soft leather armchair at a local coffee shop with a steaming mug of black coffee (zero points on my new Weight Watchers diet) and a copy of *The New York Times*. I unfolded the paper, held it up, and looked through a window at the world. The view was stunning.

The paper was rich with detail, with stories of a world I had once lived in but had been absent from for some time. I felt the greater world grabbing me through the paper. Little tentacles of connection roped me into the broader narrative of our shared existence. I felt the pain of people all over the world. I argued with myself over the positions politicians took. I challenged myself with the task of figuring out how I would solve the world's problems. And I read the opinion pieces, asking whether I agreed or disagreed with their viewpoints, and why or why not.

I had faint memories of strong opinions back when I had traveled the world and was profoundly changed by my experiences. In Kenya, I had stared my privilege in the face and wrestled with it. Flipping the pages of the newspaper, I remembered the passion I once felt for lives other than my own—the passion that had driven me to start Ugali.

After finishing my second cup of coffee and most of *The New York Times*, I drove to the Cincinnati Sports Club. It had been a long time since I had exercised. On a weekday afternoon, I hoped the facility would be nearly empty with few witnesses to my return to movement. I considered my options—weights, running the track, machines, or the pool. I had never swum laps for exercise, but I had a Speedo now and felt rather buoyant.

When I pushed off from the pool wall using the power of my legs, I tried to make myself as sleek as possible to maintain my momentum. But the water resistance soon brought me to a halt, and the struggle began.

I fought for every inch of progress across the pool, and when I made it to the other side, grabbed the wall and gasped for breath. I hung there in shock at how fatigued I was. I felt like I had just crossed the English Channel. After catching my breath, I gave myself a pep talk and headed back.

For each length, I alternated between front crawl, backstroke, breaststroke, and elementary backstroke—the last, a relaxing survival stroke. My goal was ten laps. As I swam, the countdown in my head was so loud a crowd of thousands could have been shouting it out in the slowest most undramatic fashion possible, jarring themselves awake to cheer me on as I waged the slow painful battle against lethargy. It took around twenty minutes, but I finished.

After showering, I got dressed and headed to work. It was Wednesday, the day I did the grocery shopping for the Respite Center, buying everything a fourteen-bed group house needed to fill its stomach. I also liked to buy myself a treat.

At first, it was a donut or giant cookie I ate in the car on the drive back to the center. Then some brilliant store manager decided to fill a freezer by the checkout lanes with pints of Ben & Jerry's ice cream. It was almost as if she knew I was going to get in line with my two grocery carts and realize that I had forgotten to grab my customary donut. From then on, I bought a pint of ice cream and ate the whole thing before the end of my shift.

I knew this habit and Weight Watchers diet points were incompatible. So was eating my dinner at the Respite Center.

My coworker Ernestine cooked dinner every night for the residents and she fed them well. They were either in the midst of a crisis or fresh out of one and what they needed was comfort food. That was Ernestine's specialty.

With me as her sous chef, she prepared feasts—pot roast, fried chicken, pork chops, fish cakes, meaty chili, mashed potatoes, greens in pork fat, macaroni and cheese, and green beans with butter. It was all delicious and it was for all of us—the residents, Ernestine, and me. The problem: one full plate of her food equaled more than the twenty-six Weight Watchers' points I was allotted for the entire day.

At the grocery store, as I walked along the soup aisle, a bright yellow flash caught my eye. It was a can of Old El Paso chicken tortilla soup. I picked it up, checked the nutrition information, shrugged my shoulders, and put it in my cart. Just like that, I had dinner and a special treat.

The next night, while the residents devoured their comfort food, I poured the can of soup into a bowl, microwaved it, toasted two pieces of bread, lightly brushed them with margarine, and sat down at my desk in the office for dinner. The scent of pot roast and macaroni and cheese wafted down the stairs, but strangely, I wasn't tempted.

I was excited to embark on a new adventure. I had never been on a diet before and was eager to step on the scale the following week and find out if it worked. I had to at least make it that far.

The salty broth filled my mouth. I chewed the stringy chicken and it melted away. When I swallowed, the spicy chilies did their thing. I lifted my eyebrows and looked around the office as if someone else was there eating the same thing and would share my reaction. The office was empty, so I just laughed and said to myself, "Wow, that has a kick."

I savored every molecule of my soup that night. For the first time, I didn't share the residents' dinner. Since I had started working at the Respite Center, I had taken comfort in being in a similar struggle with the residents—we had all been through some sort of mental health crisis. But with that bowl of soup, I took a step away from crisis toward health.

As the days progressed, my habits began to change. But there were setbacks—days when the enormity of the change I was taking on overwhelmed me. Each day, each step, and every morsel of food I put in my mouth was calculated and intentional. It was a huge change from microwave dinners in front of the TV, mindless snacking, and fast food. I was dismantling my life and reconstructing a new way of being.

One afternoon, overwhelmed by this task after a particularly difficult swim, I stopped at a convenience store up the hill from the gym. I walked in, bought a Krispy Kreme donut, and ate it in the car. As I licked the glaze off my fingers, my eyes watered. In that moment, the degree of change was too much. Eventually, though, even my indulgences became calculated.

It may be possible for a Cincinnatian to go three months without eating Cincinnati chili, but it rarely happens. Cincinnati chili was invented by two Macedonian immigrants, brothers Tom and John Kiradjieff, who modified a traditional Macedonian stew and began serving it over spaghetti in 1922, topped with mounds of cheddar cheese (and raw onions or beans if you so choose). They also served the chili over a small hot dog with mustard and/or onions topped with a pile of cheddar cheese: a cheese Coney.

Since then, two major chili chains have sprung up, Skyline Chili and Gold Star, along with many independent chili parlors. In the Cincinnati area, there are more than two hundred local chili parlors. They are everywhere.

Cincinnati chili is perfect for all occasions. You can feel perfectly comfortable in a chili parlor wearing a tuxedo or pajamas. While everyone is welcome, not everyone is the same. There are two types of people in a Cincinnati chili parlor: people who look at the menu and those who don't. Cincinnatians don't look at the menu. We know our order.

A few weeks into my twelve-week Weight Watchers program, I got the craving for Skyline Chili. My regular meal at Skyline was twenty-five points. However, a single cheese Coney was only eight points. I began to design a day around eating one cheese Coney. I had never ordered just one cheese Coney, and I've only seen others do it when they wind up at Skyline with friends after already eating dinner.

I went alone to the Skyline in Clifton, just three blocks from my apartment. I sat at a table by myself and ordered one cheese Coney, no mustard. While I waited, I avoided the oyster crackers in the small bowl on the table. When the Coney came, I picked up the soft bun and took a slow bite, slicing my teeth through the cheese, chili, onions, hot dog, and bun.

It was fantastic. I savored it, chewing slowly, enjoying every second. Three bites later, it was gone, and, after paying my bill, so was I. I had followed my plan perfectly. I had properly managed my craving. I was in control.

A month into my diet, Geoff called to invite me on a hike with Jon, another friend from high school. It had been a long while since I had seen my high school friends. We had hung out periodically during college, but I had drifted away from them since my diagnosis. Feeling better, I jumped at the opportunity to reconnect—unlike my college friends, they hadn't seen the full extent of my manic episode. So, I looked forward to seeing them, knowing it wouldn't trigger too many thoughts of that frightening time.

As we hiked, we reminisced about high school, those epic days filled with laughter and shenanigans. We realized our tight-knit group—Geoff, Jon, Chuck, Alan, and me—hadn't spent much time together since going off to college. Toward the end of the hike, we decided to start a hiking club to pull us all back together. Jon, in one of his signature impromptu moves, said, "And it will be called…" He pointed at me, and I blurted out the first thing that came to mind: "the Left Foot." It stuck.

Over the next three months, we quickly reestablished our tight bond during a series of three trips. In southern Indiana, we stayed at a hotel and toured a cave, firing questions at our tour guide, trying to stump him on anything cave related.

In western Indiana, we stayed in a cabin at Turkey Run State Park. During a late-night romp on the playground, Alan slipped trying to surf down an icy slide and split his chin, resulting in a late-night emergency room visit to get him stitched up.

Then, at Cumberland Falls, Kentucky, we sought out the moonbow—a rainbow created by moonlight shining through the mist of a waterfall. We didn't see it, but we laughed, and we laughed, and we laughed.

These trips were pure fun. An absolute joy. Something I hadn't experienced for a long time. Even the trip to the emergency room was high-spirited. There was a computer in the waiting room, and while Alan got his stitches, the rest of us downloaded a photoshopped image of Alan that he had previously posted on social media. His face was superimposed on Michael Jackson's picture from the cover of the *Thriller* album, the one where the King of Pop is reclined in a glowing white suit. We saved the picture as the desktop background image. Alan was almost in tears when he walked out of the treatment area and saw the computer screen. We promptly sat him in a wheelchair and rolled him out to the car.

When the Left Foot formed, I was finally on the move, but it was those trips that put a bounce in my step. Getting healthy felt good. Having fun felt great.

———

While eating Old El Paso soup, swimming laps, and reading the news, I began looking for a new job. Hoping to reignite my passion from the days before bipolar disorder, I looked for jobs in the international field. Cincinnati had few organizations doing international work and they weren't hiring. I focused my job search on Washington, DC, where my brother and Katy lived—a built-in support system if something went wrong.

My mom sent me a post from her church Listserv for a position with the Unitarian Universalist Association Washington Office for Advocacy. The job was a legislative assistant for international issues, lobbying the federal government for international intervention in Darfur, an end to the Iraq War, and funding for comprehensive HIV/AIDS prevention programs.

It was a one-year internship with the possibility of a second year. As a group, all interns met weekly with a minister for theological reflection. I would also be expected to volunteer for community organizations. It paid $28,500—$5,000 more than what I earned at the Respite Center. It sounded perfect in every way.

My mom, dad, and brother helped me put together a rèsumè and write a cover letter. I felt like I was describing someone else. No mention of bipolar disorder, even though it had consumed me since my manic episode almost two years ago. The closest my application materials came to mentioning that chapter of my life was my job at the Respite Center. I felt a bit fraudulent and worried they would ask me why I had taken a job in the mental health field after studying international affairs and doing so much work in Kenya. I wondered if I should say, "Because I was offered the job by the facilitator of my bipolar support group," or, "I needed a job, and there aren't a lot of jobs in the international field in Cincinnati?" Both true, but one truer.

I got a phone interview and Ben prepared me for it. His advice: develop three things I want them to know about me, and if I get stuck, bring the conversation to those three points. The night before my interview, we did a mock interview with Katy listening in. As I answered Ben's questions, my heart rate spiked as I spoke with urgency. I wanted to get it right. Katy gave me some tips. They both gave me encouragement. When I hung up, I knew I was as ready as I could be. My body buzzed with anticipation.

During the phone interview, I paced back and forth in the apartment I shared with Kristin, gesticulating with my hands as I answered their questions. I included all three of my points and spoke with the confidence of a man who can make his family laugh. They told me they were interviewing several candidates and would get back to me within a week.

When the 202 area code appeared on my cell phone, I jerked upright. I was in the Respite Center office, seated in the black fabric high-backed chair on wheels that I had occupied five nights a week for the last year and a half. Every shift, after serving dinner, handing out medications, and cleaning the common areas, I sat back, put my feet on the desk, and stared at the wall where a gridded dry-erase board listed all the names of the residents.

I had often wondered if my long name would fit in one of those boxes and if my life would someday lead me into a facility like this one. I had spent almost a year and a half in that chair, but when I saw the 202 number, I rocketed up the stairs to the second floor, sending it rolling backward, empty.

I stepped into the small den on the second floor, closed the door, took a deep breath, pressed the green button on my phone, and said hello.

"Adam, this is Rob Keithan from the UUA Washington Office. How are you?"

"I'm fine. How are you?"

My heart beat wildly. I thought the interview had gone well, and I wanted the job. As I hung on the edge of the future, it was clearer to me than ever that I wanted to leave Cincinnati. I wanted a fresh start, in a new city, where people didn't know my past, and hadn't seen me go manic. I wanted to stop driving past Good Samaritan Hospital feeling its shadow follow me around town. I wanted Rob to offer me the job. I wanted a ticket to a new future.

"I'm well, thanks," Rob said. "I'm calling to let you know that we've finished interviewing all the candidates for the Legislative Assistant position and we'd like to offer you the job."

I sucked in air until my lungs were bursting, "Yes!"

Rob chuckled.

"So, you'll take it?"

I was speechless. The enormity of that moment was shocking. My body vibrated with the possibility of change. Leaving Cincinnati meant a clean slate, a different world, an escape from the life bipolar disorder had designed for me. And I was ready for it. My body was healthy, my mood was stable, my mind was engaged, and my confidence was growing.

"Yes! I will take the job."

Chapter 31

FEBRUARY 19, 2023

ELY, MINNESOTA

Windswept snow covers the lake, itself a thick sheet of ice. A pack of snowmobiles shoots down the center of the lake. I come to a stop on my cross-country skis and watch them pass. The temperature is mild for a February day in northern Minnesota, but the wind brings a bite to the air. I'm out for a morning ski near Ring Rock, the lake house my mom's side of the family shares. I'm out on the lake on my own, thinking about me and the strength I once mustered.

The day before, on a walk with a friend along dirt roads and through the woods, I commented that I have high expectations of children but low expectations of adults because children are wired to grow and learn—they are compelled to develop.

"But adults only change if they have to."

I read that line in a Louise Penny novel and have repeated it many times since.

As I ski across the frozen lake, I look through the quote at myself.

When was the last time I changed?

I come around a peninsula in the lake and face an island sticking up above the ice. We call it Old Man's Island, and in the summer, we paddle there to have lunch and swim off the rocks. The wind gusts as I set off in that direction.

My past comes into focus.

In those months after the family vacation in Brazil, I changed my way of life—one of the hardest things I've done, before or since. It took tremendous grit and persistence. For a moment, I admire my past self for what I was able to accomplish those many years ago. *But was that the peak of my development? Have I changed anything since?*

I've maintained my health. I continue to eat well, exercise, and stimulate my mind. But what more have I done to be the best version of myself? My list of achievements has grown long and varied. Getting back to health allowed me to do so many things I am proud of. But have I since become any better or any healthier?

When I reach the island, I take off my skis and climb onto the rocks overlooking the lake. The island is surrounded by national forest land, a frozen expanse of trees. The wind picks up, barreling over the lake ice and hitting my body; its chill penetrates my thin layers.

An inner struggle I've managed since my diagnosis comes to the forefront of my mind— drinking.

The day before, I had three drinks in the late afternoon and woke up today feeling a little depressed. A familiar series of events. For so many years, I've known alcohol affects my moods. Hell, I heard it in my very first psychiatry session. But I've ignored that advice and tried to manage my drinking to minimize its effects. Deep down, I've always known it would be healthier to quit and that I would be more stable—and probably happier.

But whenever I thought about quitting, I would remember the carafe of wine Meredith and I shared at a bistro in Rome, the thick alluring air in the Buffalo Trace bourbon aging ware-house, and the taste of a cold beer after a long bike ride. I've told myself that I like to drink, that I don't have to give it up, and that I won't let bipolar disorder take that from me as well.

Rather than quit outright, when my mood fluctuates, I quit for a while. When I drink, I do so before dinner, so it doesn't disrupt my sleep. I've negotiated with drinking and tried to find the right spot for alcohol to fit in my life.

I close my eyes and bring my arms up to my chest, crossing them as I stand there in the wilderness. I take huge breaths, filling my lungs with cold air and feeling my body in that moment and in that place.

It hits me: stepping away from alcohol means stepping toward health. I wouldn't be leaving something behind so much as moving toward something better. I remember, truly remember, what allowed me to make all those changes years ago—a deep knowledge that I could be healthier and a profound desire to be so.

On that rock in the middle of that frozen lake, that same knowledge returns to me for the first time since. All my excuses, rationales, and resistance dissipate, and I know my days of drinking are behind me.

———

"What did drinking represent to you?" Dr. Fossum asks.

I look off to the side as if for an answer, but I can't find one. Then an image forms, a memory.

I tell Dr. Fossum about the summer after my diagno-sis—how I didn't do much beyond finish my interrupted semester, read fantasy novels, and in the afternoons, walk to the business district near my apartment, go into a bar, and drink a beer. One beer. By myself.

"It was like I was saying 'fuck you' to bipolar disorder."

I tell Dr. Fossum about my college years before my manic episode. The Budweisers and dancing until the bars closed. The nights of drinking in Kenya. So carefree. So fun. I wanted to hold onto that. And so, after my diagnosis, I kept drinking. I kept trying to hold on.

"You wanted to be a normal guy," she says. "You were hiding behind the alcohol."

I feel a release of tension as I nod.

All those years of drinking since my manic episode haven't been the same as before. There's been a voice inside my head—usually faint but sometimes blaringly loud—questioning whether I should have a drink that night, or if I should have a third, or worrying I won't sleep well because I've had too many too late.

When I've had a flare-up of my illness and stopped drinking to help stabilize my mood, as my mood improves, an inner dialogue begins along with it. *Am I well enough to drink again yet? Maybe wait another night? But I want one now, don't I?*

These thoughts have been a part of my drinking for so long that I've forgotten they weren't always there. In college, there was no inner dialogue—just the thrill of an underage beer and the welcome release of inhibitions.

Something has changed lately. I've been talking about bipolar disorder more with my family, friends, colleagues, and even my six-year-old daughter. The large role it plays in my life is becoming less of a secret. My illness doesn't frighten me as much. I'm not running or trying to escape. I just want to live with it and be as healthy as I can. Stopping drinking is an important step—a huge step—in that direction.

"I feel good," I tell Dr. Fossum. "And I don't think it's just not drinking. There's something about making the decision, about changing."

"You're choosing to be healthy," she says. "You're living more authentically. And that is amazing."

And then she asks, "Do you feel more free?"

Our eyes meet, and I smile.

Chapter 32

APRIL 30, 2006

WASHINGTON, DC

My first day at my new job was a rally organized by the Save Darfur Coalition with an expected attendance of one hundred thousand people. It would be a star-studded event—George Clooney, Olympic medalist Joey Cheek, Senator Barack Obama, Representative Nancy Pelosi, Holocaust survivor Elie Wiesel, and Reverend Al Sharpton would all take the stage.

The National Mall was empty early that Sunday morning, but it would soon be packed. The Capitol Building rose up in front of me, the Washington Monument behind, with the stage erected on the long grassy strip between them.

The morning sun hit my face as I headed toward the gathering spot for the Unitarian Universalists (or UUs as we call ourselves) coming to the rally. We would meet each other, hear from some Darfuri refugees, and eat snacks before walking together to the main rally.

The UUs weren't as thirsty as we had anticipated. Six two-gallon water jugs remained when our gathering ended, and everyone marched toward the main rally. Meredith, my fellow intern, and I grabbed two jugs and a sleeve of plastic cups and hustled to catch up with the procession.

The temperature hovered just below seventy degrees during the four-hour rally, but there was no protection from the sun on the National Mall. About an hour into the rally, Meredith and I began moving through the crowd with the water. Weaving our way through, we yelled out like vendors at a baseball game, "Free water here, get your water."

At first, people were tentative, perhaps even suspicious of these strangers offering what they claimed was water. But, as the afternoon wore on and the sun continued to arc over the huddled masses, attitudes changed. Someone stopped us, took a cup, and we poured a drink. Before the pour was finished, two or three other people grabbed cups and waited their turn. Eventually, we ran out of cups and poured water directly into people's mouths.

Meredith and I approached our task with joy. It felt good to have a purpose in the crowd of thousands. We were hydrating the movement.

By the time we ran out of water and turned back to the program, the crowd was thinning, and the rally was coming to an end. After George Clooney spoke, Meredith and I decided that it was time to quench our own thirst. It was time to find a bar.

We walked past the stage, climbed Capitol Hill, and found a table on the front patio of Union Pub, on Massachusetts Avenue. From the moment we left the rally until we finished a pitcher of frozen margaritas (Meredith claims they were daiquiris), we never stopped chattering.

Everything I learned about her made me want to know more, and the feeling seemed mutual. We talked about college, studying abroad, Minnesota, and our families. I asked her about her long-distance relationship, hoping to learn more about how to handle mine. We laughed about brain freeze. The conversation was playful. We jumped between topics and time like two children hopping rocks along a coastline.

When I finally checked the time, I realized I was running late to a meeting with my new landlord, so we paid, said our see-you-tomorrows, and I ran off toward the Metro. I floated through the city. I smiled and enjoyed the sensation of carrying what appeared to be a lighter load. In one day, I had done something meaningful for others and made a new friend.

Kristin came to visit for a long July Fourth weekend. We went camping in Shenandoah National Park. From the moment she arrived, there was tension between us.

When I took the job in DC, our plan was to stay together, maintain our love despite the distance, and after a year I would return to Cincinnati. The job posting had said the position was for one year, with the possibility of a second year. But when I started, I learned that the position was almost guaranteed to be two years. This changed things.

While we hiked through the mountains, Kristin looked for certainty; she wanted to know when we would reunite. She proposed moving to DC, which I didn't encourage. I was in love with my new life and nervous her presence would change that. She wanted me to commit to returning to Cincinnati after a year, but I wanted to keep my options open.

On the last day of her visit, we climbed Old Rag, the most popular hike in the region. We climbed the mountain largely in silence. When Kristin boarded her flight back to Cincinnati, nothing was settled—we were together, but far apart.

A month later, Meredith and I climbed Old Rag. We had discovered we both liked hiking, so I took her to the best trail I knew. From the moment I picked her up early in the morning, we talked nonstop until I dropped her off late in the evening.

It was an epic hike. We stumbled across a black bear, terrifying us, and sending us running through the forest. We came across a rattlesnake in the middle of the trail. At the end of the hike, we even went for a little dip in a shallow creek. Also, I ate a plum.

It was my first plum. As a youngster, I was a very picky eater—a terrible eater. When it came to fruit, I ate only grapes, watermelon, and apples. Plums were out of the question.

By the time I moved to DC, my palate had expanded, largely thanks to international travel, but each expansion was still fear-inducing. When Meredith discovered I had never eaten a plum, she looked at me like I was a different species. She handed me one from her packed lunch, and I tore into it with the levity the moment warranted.

It was delicious.

When its skin broke and the soft flesh hit my tongue, I smiled at Meredith, and she giggled. She had grown up in a home where fruit was served with every meal. Plums were nothing to her, but she took joy in my discovery. I didn't eat the plum daintily; I ravished it. I was ready for something new.

Toward the end of our hike, Meredith went to pee in the woods, and I turned and looked back up the trail. I remembered hiking it with Kristin just the month before and couldn't help but compare it with my unfolding adventure with Meredith. It was like I was walking a different trail.

As Meredith came out of the woods, the truth struck me: it wasn't going to work with Kristin. Just like that, my feelings changed, and my love for Kristin faded. I hadn't fallen in love with Meredith yet, but I had fallen in love with plums, and there was no going back.

***

The truth I recognized on that hike wasn't liberating; it was terrifying.

My fear confused me, at first; then, it turned me into a coward. *Maybe I was wrong*, I thought. Kristin had been so wonderful to me. She had supported me through my darkest hours. She had been loving and nurturing. She had been the best part of my last two years. How could I abandon her now that things were going well for me?

I had loved her so much—from the very first time we met. She was beautiful, different, and strong. She was fierce. But she anchored me in a past I wanted to escape.

I wrestled with these questions, thinking myself into confusion. I talked to my brother and sister. Finally, I called my mom.

She listened as I poured out my confusion. As I spoke, I listened to myself. I could hear that I wasn't truly confused. No, I was just trying to hide from the truth. And as I spoke, the truth just got clearer. Yes, Kristin and I had been through a lot together. She had been wonderful to me. I would always feel indebted to her. I would always feel like I could have been better to her. But it was over. I wasn't in love with her anymore. There was no way to hide from that.

When I finished talking, my mom was quiet. She didn't need to say anything. Just by making the call, I was finally facing the truth.

When my mom finally spoke, the words weren't all that important; it was her tone. Her cadence was smooth and steady. There was no surprise in her voice. She spoke reflectively as if she had been anticipating this conversation for months. She spoke with understanding. She knew why it was difficult for me, for Kristin, and for anyone in our situation. She understood better than I did. But she knew I understood enough.

"Adam, I think you just need to listen to yourself."

Kristin and I had been having loaded conversations over the past week, ever since I returned from my hike with Meredith. She was frustrated and I was infuriating her. One day I would tell her she was the most important thing in the world to me; the next day I didn't want to talk.

Kristin had loved me through my worst times. Without her, where would I turn if I needed a safe place? No one in Washington knew what I had been through. Not even Ben and Katy. They hadn't been there as I forced myself out of bed every morning. They hadn't held my hand while I cried on my balcony. No one in Washington knew how deep my depression had been and how terrified I was of going back there.

In my darkest hours, Kristin had kept me safe and helped me stay alive. Even then, when Washington was too big for me and I felt small and vulnerable, I would call her. She would comfort me, and I would feel like everything would be okay. Without her, who would I call when the demons of my past haunted my present?

Ending our relationship was an extremely difficult thing to do. I was twenty-four years old. I had never been in a relationship as long-lasting, never lived with a girlfriend before, never moved away from a great love, and never broken up with a woman whose life had become so entwined with mine.

A few days after talking to my mom, I paced in my small Washington bedroom as Kristin told me she couldn't wait on me any longer. She needed control of her life, and she wouldn't allow me to treat her the way I was. She cut me loose. It wasn't that she loved me less or wanted to be rid of me. I think she saw me looking out the window, longing to leave my past behind, yearning for freedom but too scared to grab it. And she had mercy.

Two weeks after breaking up on the phone, I flew to Cincinnati for Labor Day weekend. Kristin and I met in a park three blocks from her apartment. Even though we had already broken up on the phone, we had agreed it couldn't end that way. We needed to see each other in person one more time. I handed her a letter. She read it. We cried. We hugged. And kissed. Then, I asked her to get my television from her apartment.

We followed a trail out of the park and walked to her apartment building, the same one we had lived in together for ten months. We climbed the wide stairs and went into her apartment. I unplugged the television and slung the cord up over the top while Kristin stood there sobbing. The huge television was hard for one man to carry, but I stretched my arms around it, hoisted it up, and walked out the door with my heavy load, alone.

Chapter 33

MARCH 17, 2023
St. Paul, Minnesota

Once again, the mail has come and there's nothing from Kristin. Every day for the last few months, when I've collected the mail, I've hoped for a response to my letter. I've told myself many stories about why she hasn't replied. I imagine my letter opened, sitting on her desk, waiting for her to find the right words. I wonder if my internet sleuthing yielded the wrong address.

But what I picture most is Kristin picking my letter from her stack of mail, seeing my name in the return address, and dropping it in the recycling bin.

Why did I write?

Do I have a patronizing desire to make sure she is okay? Am I guilt-ridden from leaving her behind when I left Cincinnati, ultimately leading to the end of our relationship? Do I just miss her being in my life?

I'm subbing in a Montessori classroom with twenty young children when Kristin comes to mind again. The students eat lunch peacefully, scooping pasta out of thermoses with small utensils, and slowly chewing carrot sticks. There's nothing to do but watch them and occasionally help open a food container, so my mind wanders. For the first time, I wonder, *What do I want Kristin to say?*

I exhale as that question brings everything into focus.

I want her to tell me she is fine—that she really is. That what happened between us is in the past, and she has moved on and holds no bad feelings. That what we shared was special, and she looks back on it kindly and with understanding. I want her to be happy for me, for the things I've accomplished, and for the ways I've grown.

Finally, I realize what I want most of all: I want her to forgive me.

I see what was lacking in the letter I wrote. I never apologized.

I told myself I didn't have anything to apologize for. It's been so long that the details of my shortcomings are fuzzy—and what would a generalized "I'm sorry" even mean? But this isn't true. There's one vivid memory that keeps running through my mind, and I know it captures the essence of my mistreatment of her.

More than a year after my manic episode, Kristin and I took a trip to the Boundary Waters Canoe Area Wilderness in northern Minnesota, my favorite place on earth. It was the summer I became the "Edging Man." My confidence was boosted, and while I hadn't started Lamictal yet, my mood was more stable than it had been at any point since my diagnosis.

The Boundary Waters is a vast expanse of lakes only accessible by canoe. Where one lake ends, paddlers shoulder their gear-filled backpacks, flip their canoes onto their shoulders, and portage everything to the next lake. Sometimes the portages are ten feet, sometimes they're over a mile.

I had done many canoe trips in my life, but this was Kristin's first. Eager to conquer the first portage and show off my talent at carrying a canoe, I loaded her up with two hefty packs—one on her back and one on her front. I put on a daypack, flipped the canoe onto my shoulders, and set off down the trail. It was a long portage, around a mile. As I marched along, sweat beginning to form, and mosquitoes buzzed around my face. I felt strong and proud. When I reached the end, I rolled the canoe off my shoulders and into the lake, propped it up on shore, and waited for Kristin. After a couple minutes, I got concerned and walked back down the trail.

When I finally found her, she was in tears. The two giant packs had been an enormous load for her narrow frame, and she had to drop one beside the trail and leave it. She was in pain; she felt like a failure; and I had left her behind.

Sitting among those peaceful children, I realize why I wrote to her.

Yes, I miss her and want to connect. But I'm also a guilt-ridden ex-boyfriend who wants to be forgiven.

On that portage and then later, when I left Cincinnati, I was so focused on myself—on reconnecting with the strength I once had and on moving forward without looking back—that I forgot about her and the weight I had put on her shoulders.

Back at home after the school day ends, I search my old computer files to find the letter I gave to her in the park the last time we saw each other. As I read it, parts make me cringe and parts make me smile. The conclusion does both.

"I know that I have hurt you. For that, I ask your forgiveness. I know that I have loved you. Of that, I will always be proud. As you move forward and encounter new challenges, new joys, and new sorrows, or if you wish to revisit the memories I am sure we will both cherish, please know that I'm here. I'm here."

Two truths and a lie.

I do want forgiveness. I am still proud of having loved her. But "I'm here" was bullshit.

When I wrote that letter, I was running away, and only now am I looking back. She may have stopped looking back a long time ago.

This time I email. And this time I say I'm sorry.

Chapter 34

SEPTEMBER 15, 2023

St. Paul, Minnesota

I lean back on Dr. Fossum's couch, stretch my left arm out on the backrest, and smile. "I'm doing good," I say.

This has been my initial report for a few sessions now. I haven't cried for a long while, and I have a feeling—which has grown all summer—that this chapter of therapy is ending.

She notices I'm wearing a Minnesota "Up North" hoodie—a change from the Cincinnati sweatshirts I wore all winter. Yes, I tell her, I'm trying to explore my new home more, find the places I love, settle in, and enjoy myself.

Over the summer, when I wasn't focused on caring for Phoenix, my personal goal was to decide whether to go back into the classroom as an assistant in a regular part-time role. After many conversations with Meredith and an honest self-assessment, I chose to be a homemaker this school year. Failing as a lead teacher wounded me and grieving our move depleted me.

What I need now is to keep building myself back up. I'm not ready to learn a new job—and open the door to potential failure. I want to enjoy myself, have fun, and be a healthier father and husband. Plus, Meredith has gotten used to the pleasures of having a homemaker as a spouse:

the fridge is magically filled with groceries, dinner appears on the table, and weekends are filled with fun rather than chores.

In the last couple of sessions, Dr. Fossum and I have talked about suspending therapy. We haven't agreed on when that will happen, but as our conversation flows, I get the sense today is the day. It's hard to justify the therapy bill when I'm mostly reporting good news or challenges I've handled on my own. At a deeper level, I know there is only so much personal transformation I can endure at one time. I'm sure there is a lot more I can work on, but for now, I've done enough.

I have finally faced all the pain, fear, and sorrow I've hidden from and carried around in silence since I left Cincinnati seventeen years ago. I've loved and forgiven myself for hitting my mother. I've embraced myself as I fought the restraints in the hospital. I've listened to and trusted myself as I contemplated suicide on my balcony. I've tried to make amends with Patrick and Kristin.

Those painful moments no longer hurt. Remembering them will always be emotional, but there is a difference between emotion and pain.

Recently, when I've felt hypomania coming on, a roughening settling in, or a slumping sadness, I haven't retreated to my room and distracted myself from a growing panic that the worst might be happening again. I'm no longer scared of going back because I've done that now, and while the journey brought many tears, it has allowed me to be bipolar today without the fear of being bipolar as I was.

I'm not sure how often I'll tell the stories from those two years when bipolar disorder was so dominant in my life, but now I know how to tell them—with kindness, forgiveness, and understanding. They aren't horror stories. They are human stories.

At the close of our session, Dr. Fossum and I don't schedule another.

"If you need me," she says, "get in touch."

I take a deep breath and look into her eyes. "Thank you."

As I approach the door, I think back to the first time I walked through it a year ago.

Distraught.

Looking for a way forward.

I wasn't expecting to look back—definitely not as far back as I have—and I certainly didn't think that is where I would find my way forward.

Walking home, I remember the question Dr. Fossum asked me in our first session—*Was leaving Cincinnati a good thing for you?*

Suddenly, I remember how I felt on the drive from Cincinnati to Washington, DC. My car packed with my belongings. My fingers drumming the steering wheel. A knot that had been tied around my life for two years loosened with every mile I put behind me.

The feeling of that moment returns to me, and it is familiar, a sensation I've felt a lot recently.

Freedom.

I felt free.

A fresh start was what I needed then, and the only way I knew how to get it was by leaving.

A fresh start is what I have now, and the only way I could claim it was by going back.

Epilogue

I once thought I had figured out how to achieve balance and thrive while living with bipolar disorder.

An earlier version of this book was potentially titled *Bipolar and Balanced* or *Because of Love: How I Learned to Thrive While Living with Bipolar Disorder*. I felt I had figured out how to manage bipolar disorder, and I wanted to share the lessons I learned with others.

I thought the keys were to get enough sleep, eat well, exercise, take medications, seek out professional help when needed, and, if shit got rough, retreat and give it time.

These lessons were valuable and hard-won.

To get good sleep, I've tried many things over the years—meditation, sound machines, antianxiety pills, sleeping pills, and a sleep therapist.

My diet is tied to my moods. When I'm in a funk, I go back for seconds and snack aggressively, ensuring that my weight has never been stable. I've often informally returned to calorie consciousness to help shed the after-effects of a bipolar roughening.

I've also continued exercising since those first laps in the pool. For many years, I swam laps, then started running, and now I mostly bike and walk.

My commitment to my medications has never wavered. My regimen has rarely changed over the years, but during times of persistent instability, I've swapped pills or changed dosages.

When I've needed professional help, I've cast a wide net, gaining insight and healing from talk therapists, ministers, psychics, and a shaman.

And when I've recognized my mood spiraling out of control, I've gathered my comfort foods, a streaming device, and a good novel and barricaded myself in my room until I felt better.

As I set out to write the first draft of this book ten years ago, I thought this recipe for wellness was worth sharing. Today, I see it differently. Yes, all those things are vital at times, but they are more of a chapter than a book.

In the last year, since I abruptly left my job as a lead teacher and struggled to regain my equilibrium, my concept of wellness expanded beyond my prior field of vision.

Wellness is talking to Meredith about my moods, my attempts to manage them, and what she can do to help. During times of instability, wellness is negotiating with Meredith about what social engagements I should show up for and what I can skip.

Wellness is writing out a list of best intentions or rules—for my daily life and for making big decisions—then sharing the list with Meredith and incorporating what we can into our family rhythm. Wellness is struggling through depression on the couch in the living room in the presence of my wife and daughter rather than hiding away in my bedroom.

Wellness is talking about bipolar disorder in my job interviews. Wellness is being fully present when Phoenix gets off the school bus and begins telling me about her day. Wellness is honoring each phase of my life and doing my best to be in good relationships with all the people important to me. Wellness is learning how to grieve.

And that's just the beginning of a list without end.

I've had an exceptional feeling recently that I can only describe as peace. My mind is sharp but settled; I'm content just listening. I'm full of forgiveness and understanding, both of myself and others. I have a ready laugh, and I'm filled with a steady energy from morning to night.

This state of being sometimes lasts only a short while but has begun stretching out for days or even weeks. What's brought this on has been that familiar focus on my internal well-being coupled with my newfound efforts to strengthen my bonds with the world around me.

The latter part has a lot to do with my new openness about bipolar disorder. It's no longer something I stay quiet about, nor is it something I interject needlessly. I just talk about it when it's on my mind and seems relevant. And I've learned it's often on my mind and relevant.

This has always been the case, but until recently, I stayed silent and hid. And when things got rough, I even tried to hide from myself. Now, though, I'm limiting the role distraction plays in my life. As I do, my whole life comes into focus.

Wellness isn't something I will achieve. But I can always hope to get well.

That hope comes through long and open conversations with loved ones, making choices that honor my limitations, taking risks by changing long-established patterns, seeking out passions that meaningfully connect me to the world, being thoughtful in how I love the people in my life, and having faith that I am okay.

Even when I'm in pain and life is difficult, I am okay.

Acknowledgments

Every person who I mention in this book made it possible, especially Meredith, who always cultivated the space in our family life when I returned to this project and immersed myself in it. She trusted what I was doing was important, even though ten years passed between the two drafts I shared with her. Eric Larson coached me through my first draft. Greg Kornbluh and Jie Wronski-Riley gave transformative feedback on my third draft. Sharon Dittmar and Alice Connor, my writing pals, provided crucial encouragement. Ellen Akins was the editor I needed to shape the manuscript. And Jo Bartlett was the editor I needed to hone it. Ramsey Ford's cover art nailed it. Rabbi Adam Spilker blessed the manuscript, giving me peace of mind as I first sent it to others. And finally, a big thank-you to my daughter, Phoenix, for inspiring the title and inspiring me.

9 7 9 8 8 8 6 7 9 5 1 9 6